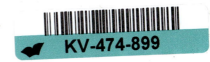

HIV and AIDS Care

HIV and AIDS Care

Practical Approaches

Edited by Louise Cusack and Surinder Singh

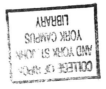
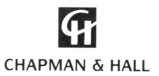

CHAPMAN & HALL

London · Glasgow · Weinheim · New York · Tokyo · Melbourne · Madras

Published by Chapman & Hall, 2–6 Boundary Row, London SE1 8HN, UK

Chapman & Hall, 2–6 Boundary Row, London SE1 8HN, UK

Blackie Academic & Professional, Wester Cleddens Road, Bishopbriggs, Glasgow G64 2NZ, UK

Chapman & Hall GmbH, Pappelallee 3, 69469 Weinheim, Germany

Chapman & Hall Inc., One Penn Plaza, 41st Floor, New York NY 10119, USA

Chapman & Hall Japan, Thomson Publishing Japan, Hirakawacho Nemoto Building, 6F, 1–7–11 Hirakawa-cho, Chiyoda-ku, Tokyo 102, Japan

Chapman & Hall Australia, Thomas Nelson Australia, 102 Dodds Street, South Melbourne, Victoria 3205, Australia

Chapman & Hall India, R. Seshadri, 32 Second Main Road, CIT East, Madras 600 035, India

Distributed in the USA and Canada by Singular Publishing Group Inc., 4284 41st Street, San Diego, California 92105

First edition 1994

© 1994 Chapman & Hall

Phototypeset in Times by Intype, London

Printed in Great Britain by St Edmundsbury Press, St Edmunds, Bury

ISBN 0 412 45940 X   (PB) 1 56593 144 0 (USA)

A catalogue record for this book is available from the British Library

Library of Congress Catalog Card Number: 93–74439

Printed on permanent acid-free text paper, manufactured in accordance with ANSI/NISO Z39.48–1992 and ANSI/NISO Z39.48–1984 (Permanence of Paper).

Contents

Foreword

Immunodeficiency due to the human immunodeficiency virus is a chronic multisystem disease. It is also a disease which causes physical, social and psychological morbidity. Additionally, more and more people with immunodeficiency are living longer and spending more time in the community. Therefore, in order to maximize their potential for good quality life many different skills need to be utilized. For this reason a multidisciplinary approach is fundamental to the planning and provision of services to those affected.

The editors of this book have many years of experience of caring for people with HIV infection, including multidisciplinary work, discharge planning, staff support and voluntary sector liaison in such diverse settings as hospice, day unit and hospital. They are ideally placed to give a broad view of the range of needs of people with HIV.

This book will give confidence to those professionals who are called upon to give advice and help to people with HIV disease but who may not have a wide clinical experience of the syndrome. It will provide support and guidance to all the members of the multidisciplinary team and help them to utilize their pre-existing skills in ways that are appropriate for this new and challenging client-group.

Dr S.J. Mansfield
Consultant Physician

Acknowledgements

Many people have contributed to the writing of this book and we would like to thank them for their hard work and valuable contribution.

We would also like to thank Brian and Thomas Cusack and Lucy Reilly who supported and encouraged us and gave us without complaint, time to work and write. A special thanks must go to our respective families for their help and encouragement.

A special mention must be extended to Dr Simon Mansfield who, although not directly involved in the book, contributed so much. He died in April 1993.

Finally our thanks go to all those individuals with chronic HIV infection or AIDS, who, in sharing their experience with us, have taught us much.

1

Introduction

Surinder Singh and Louise Cusack

At the conclusion of events such as this one, we find there is
more in which we are alike than different.

Albert Camus, **The Plague**

1981 will go down in medical history as a very significant year. It
was in that year that a new condition revealed itself to be infectious, transmissible and above all, often fatal.

Ten years on, the acronym A.I.D.S., which translates as the
Acquired Immune Deficiency Syndrome, reflects that much has
changed in our understanding of the condition. In addition our
knowledge is still rapidly changing and every day new challenges
are facing health care workers world-wide as a direct consequence
of AIDS and its various complications.

Since 1981, a remarkable amount of research data has been
accumulated about the virus, its transmission and its effects. What
has become clear is that chronic HIV infection and AIDS are not
merely medical diagnoses but rather complex conditions with
often serious complications. These complications are sometimes
physical, sometimes psychological, and at other times social. More
often than not, it is a combination of these problems which results
in an individual consulting a health care professional.

In a multisystem disorder like HIV infection, various professionals can be involved and it is a measure of the success of
these working groups which ultimately determines whether need
is met or not. One of the themes of this book is that successful
collaboration and coordination of various professionals is the key
to providing quality care.

The editors of the book believe that although HIV infection
with AIDS is relatively new, many of the challenges have been
encountered before in general medicine, psychiatry, primary care
and palliative care. Nevertheless, the severity of morbidity in HIV

infection, the relative youth of those affected and the misconceptions which surround the condition make the task of caring that much harder. We believe that one of the strategies that may be adopted to overcome these dangerous misconceptions is to 'normalize' HIV infection and AIDS, that is, treat it like other chronic conditions.

People with such conditions often require specialist help and need extra support at home in a way which is professional, coordinated, and tailored to each individual. Clinicians help to define needs, and support therapists enable people to live quality lives. Treatment for those with HIV infection and AIDS ought to be no different in this respect. The increasing emphasis on care in the community also means that more therapists will be meeting people affected by AIDS, often for the first time.

It is with these ideals that we have produced this book for non-specialists and specialists alike. We would be thrilled to know if it has proved useful especially for those with limited experience of the condition since then it will have fulfilled its aims.

AIMS OF THIS BOOK

A holistic approach to care of people with chronic HIV infection and AIDS means that a number of professionals have much to contribute. The aims of this book are:

- To provide information for therapists to ensure that chronic HIV infection and AIDS is regarded as other chronic conditions requiring a balanced response to care involving community, as well as hospital resources to meet need.
- To ensure that a multidisciplinary approach to care is highlighted and emphasized as a good working model, designed to benefit those with chronic HIV infection.
- To emphasize the multifaceted role of the specialist therapists in the overall care of individuals with chronic HIV infection and AIDS. Palliative care is highlighted as an example [1].

Unfortunately it is beyond the remit of this book to address paediatric issues although the aims above would be as relevant (if not more so) to this group of individuals. Where appropriate, case studies will be presented to highlight specific points.

This book contains chapters written by a broad range of practitioners and therapists. Each of these provide a unique insight into their specific therapeutic roles and responsibilities. This introductory chapter is designed to set the scene with the aims of the text and a description of the global position of HIV infection and AIDS. One recurring theme throughout the book is the importance of communication and thus it rightly appears in the first chapter. Chapter 2 is a comprehensive medical account of HIV infection with a description of its pathogenesis. The complications of HIV infection are also described along with treatment regimes. The central four chapters of the book, Chapters 3–6, represent occupational therapy, physiotherapy, dietetics and social work. The four practitioners describe their different perspectives, each individual and complementary to each other. Chapter 7 has been written by a person with HIV infection. His personal, sometimes poignant, but always compelling account provides an important counterbalance to the previous chapters. The important case history of A.S. is described in chapter 8. Here many of the themes of the book are pulled together in what was a complex and intricate case. Concepts such as adjustment to illness, discharge planning and purposeful team working in order to meet the patient's expectations and needs are fully described. Because A.S. did become quite ill following a period of stabilization, the end stages of his condition are highlighted. A section on palliative care follows. The appendix is a compendium of common medication regimes and there is a bibliography at the end of the book.

A GLOBAL PERSPECTIVE

Initially, and certainly in the West, many of those infected with HIV were gay men. This client-group were largely responsible for a well-motivated, sensitive and galvanized movement to modify behaviour and establish support systems for those diagnosed as HIV positive and who had AIDS. What has been called the 'second wave' of those affected is increasingly manifest in the developed countries, that is, women (and children) and those infected heterosexually.

World-wide, approximately 75% of all infections have been sexually transmitted, with a heterosexual to homosexual ratio of about 7:1. In addition, of all the world's HIV infected adults, just over a third are women and the female to male ratio is increasing rapidly. The continued and sustained rise in the number of women affected inevitably translates into rising numbers of HIV/AIDS-affected orphans with an immeasurable toll of suffering and morbidity.

Already some countries in Africa reveal frighteningly high prevalence rates for HIV infection with potentially devastating results for the socio-economic welfare of the country. For example, the prevalence of HIV infection among men attending a sexually-transmitted disease clinic in Nairobi has increased eightfold in just ten years [2]. In South-East Asia the volatility of the pandemic becomes all too clear when considering that in a few vital years the numbers infected have risen to over ten times that of Britain.

It is not surprising that HIV infection has been identified as the greatest public health challenge facing the human population. Resources to meet this global pandemic are clearly not evenly distributed, and some of the countries just mentioned are the least able to withstand such a burden on their own already faltering health care systems.

Many reasons exist as to why HIV/AIDS is the subject of prejudice and discrimination. Unfortunately the response by some authorities has been extremely negative, and evidence exists for clear breaches of human rights, purely on account of a person's HIV status.

Dr Jonathan Mann – Director of the International AIDS Centre at Harvard University in the US, speaks about the interrelationship of human rights and public health which is 'one of the great advances in the history of health and society' [3]. He sees the collective response to the epidemic as a catalyst leading to a revolution in health. Human rights are vital for HIV prevention; discrimination and stigma create conditions which encourage perpetuation of the disease, by causing social marginalization and therefore leading to lack of the social, economic and political power which people need to protect themselves [4].

The issue of a uniform and consistent, world-wide response to HIV infection and AIDS comes to the fore. The availability of drugs (antibiotics, antiretroviral agents) and access to health care are just two parameters which will vary enormously depending on where an individual lives. A global response is the imperative for such a global condition.

CARE STRUCTURES AND COMMUNICATION

In Britain many patients with AIDS spend less and less time in hospital, compared with previously when protracted stays were frequent. The greater emphasis on out-patient care means that many patients spend 80% of time at home, following a diagnosis of AIDS, rather than in hospital or other care institutions.

World-wide (that is, where choices exist) there is a shift away from institutional and residential care. In Britain, greater emphasis is placed on community care. For example whereas previously, diagnosis and management of pneumocystis pneumonia always took place within hospitals (Chapter 2), now certain groups of patients with this pneumonia can be treated as out-patients [5].

An essential prerequisite, if this trend is to be sustained, is the placement, availability and effectiveness of support in the communities in which patients normally reside. Ultimately it is the success of these supporting resources which will determine whether continued management can take place in the community or in hospital.

In Britain the two arms of the National Health Service, that is, primary and secondary care, are complementary. Thus while the focus is on providing care at home, a deteriorating condition or the need for further investigations may necessitate hospital care.

Routine out-patient care can be carried out by general practitioners (GPs) so long as there is good communication between hospital and general practitioner. Unfortunately because this relationship is not seen to be important by some and thus neglected, patients lose out in times of crises or during the terminal phase of the illness when home care is seen to be a priority. There is certainly evidence that for this aspect of care many individuals are forced to spend their last days in institutions including hospitals when their preference is to be at home [6].

Though the reasons why this happens is beyond the remit of this chapter, all hospital care workers have an important role in ensuring that the patient is given as much information as possible in order to register him with a local general practitioner or primary care physician. Hospitals, of course fulfil a vital function and have roles to play in research, education and the provision of acute care. It is a particular strength in Britain that the complement of primary and secondary care can work so well, can provide an efficient service and is relatively cost-effective [7].

The communication which is so vital between care structures is also equally important at the level of primary care. A fully effective team within primary care needs the full services of the district nurse, occupational therapist, physiotherapist, as well as liaison nurses and physicians to ensure need is met. Team meetings or planning meetings are necessary to ensure that supervision and guidance is maintained, investigation and re-assessments continue, and follow-up arranged.

Where a higher level of care is needed, other support can be mobilized – care assistants, volunteers from various agencies and help from social services. It is important to note that the best co-ordinator for all these carers is the individual himself, though clearly this is not always possible, feasible or desirable.

One factor which many cite within the health care community is the lack of training and education which they have received in the overall care of patients with chronic HIV infection and AIDS. Over ten years have elapsed since the original infection came to light and there is little excuse for total ignorance. The wide range of contributors to this book is a reflection of our collective belief that a multidisciplinary approach to patient care is the most effective. We hope this book will provide useful, practical information, engage intellectual minds and above all encourage others to adopt a similar approach.

The ever-present problem of writing about patients as 'he' or 'she' is one we have not solved. We have sided with convention and use 'he' or 'him' throughout this book even though many of the individuals concerned are women. We are deeply committed to equal opportunities in all aspects of health care, indeed in all walks of life, and find prejudice and discrimination based upon sex, creed, religion, ability, race, culture and sexual orientation abhorrent.

It is prudent to mention here the views of Ivor Lyford, the author of Chapter 7, on language. He states that language is just as important as services: terms such as 'AIDS victim', 'AIDS sufferer' or 'AIDS carrier' are demeaning and disempowering. It is preferable to speak of who he *is*, that is, a *person* with HIV infection or a *person* with AIDS. Terms such as 'victim' imply that there is a judgment of innocence or guilt on the person with HIV/AIDS. Ivor clearly states that nobody wanted or invited HIV into their lives, and thus all of those affected are equally deserving of care and respect. We, the editors, wholeheartedly support this view. Where possible we have tried our best to write with the above in mind, however it is the responsibility of the editors if this does not hold true throughout the book.

The community response to AIDS has taught us at least four reasons to promote human rights and dignity: first, because it is right to do so: second, because preventing discrimination helps ensure a more effective HIV prevention programme; third, because social marginalization intensifies the risk of HIV penetration into and spread within societies; and fourth, because the capacity of a community to respond to AIDS is an expression of the basic right of people to participate in decisions which affect them.

Dr Jonathan Mann
Director, International AIDS Centre, Harvard, USA
Second International NGO Conference
November 1991

Surinder Singh
Louise Cusack

REFERENCES

1. Wild, L., Phillips, P. and Singh, S. (1990) The role of the Occupational Therapist in HIV disease and AIDS. *British Journal of Occupational Therapy*, **53**(5), 181–4.
2. Mann, J. *AIDS in the 1990s: A global analysis*, Lecture at The Royal Society of Health, London, 28 April 1992.
3. ibid.
4. Lucas, S. (1991) Policies for Solidarity: A personal view of the second international conference for NGOs working on AIDS. *AIDS CARE*, **3**, 89–101.
5. Youle, M., Clarbour, J., Wade, P. *AIDS: Therapeutics in HIV disease*. Churchill Livingstone, Edinburgh, 1988, pp. 11–27.
6. Kennedy, A., Ellam, G.A., Porter, J.D.H. *Where are people in England and Wales dying from AIDS?*, Poster presentation, 5th International Conference on AIDS 1989, Montreal, Canada (Poster TH.E.P.47).
7. Pinching, A. (1989) Models of clinical care. *AIDS*, **3** (supplement): S209–S213.

2

A medical perspective

Surinder Singh

AIDS is the acronym for the **Acquired Immune Deficiency Syndrome**, a condition representing the most serious and often fatal illness resulting from the **Human Immune Deficiency Virus (HIV)**. HIV was identified in 1983 as the infectious agent responsible for many of the symptoms with illnesses associated with AIDS though previously it had been called HTLV–111 (Human T-Lymphotropic Virus) or LAV (Lymphadenopathy-Associated Virus).

WHAT IS A VIRUS?

A **virus**, of which there are hundreds and thousands, is an organism or microbe which is far more basic than any bacterial organism. In fact without a 'host' a virus is relatively inert and therefore dependent on the host cell for replication and overall viability.

Fundamental to all viruses is their ability to enter living cells and 'take command' of the functions of the cell, influencing them to synthesize new virus particles. Many of the harmful effects of a virus are due to the direct invasion of the host cells. In contrast, bacteria can produce toxins as well as invade locally in order to exert their harmful effects.

Technically therefore, a virus is highly parasitic, being dependent on the host and inducing damage. Structurally it consists of a shell, usually protein and called a **capsid**, surrounding a single molecule of nucleic acid (either RNA or DNA). Sometimes an outer membrane exists, called an **envelope**, which is partially derived from the host cell's outer coating on entry into the cell. Viruses are much smaller than bacteria and can only be viewed through an electron microscope.

HIV INFECTION

An investigation of the cellular process involving HIV is not an integral part of this book; however, a brief description will be given in order to facilitate understanding.

A specific target of HIV within the human body is a subset of the lymphocytes in the immune system. The **lymphocytes** are part of the white cells in blood and can be found in circulation in most organs of the body (the other white cell constituents are neutrophils and granulocytes). The lymphocytes most affected are called **T helper/inducer cells** or **CD4 cells**, because of the name given to the receptor (CD4 molecule) which appears to attract the HIV to the host cell. It is this attraction which profoundly affects the overall function of the body's immunity to counteract infections and thus leaves the body vulnerable to an array of infections and infestations. Many believe that HIV slowly but progressively destroys these T-cells over many months and years and ultimately leaves the body immune deficient. There are other systems within the body which are affected, specifically the gastro-intestinal system, respiratory system and perhaps most worryingly the nervous system.

It is postulated, that once acquired, the infection is lifelong, though the person infected may not develop symptoms for an extended period (the so-called latent period). Even though individuals may remain asymptomatic, they are potentially infectious to others, and hence it is vital to stress this point in any preventative health programme within the sphere of HIV and AIDS. The only sure way of remaining safe from HIV infection and AIDS is through primary prevention, one of the areas which should be covered by counselling and education. An example of primary prevention education is to publicize that individuals who are unknowingly HIV positive can transmit the virus through unsafe sex or sharing needles.

Rapid advances in our base line knowledge have been made in the past ten years but many uncertainties surround the above processes. Factors which may trigger symptoms in an individual with chronic HIV infection are yet unknown, as are the exact mechanisms through which the virus exerts its destructive effect. Continued work is needed to explore further changes in the virus itself as well as other related and equally harmful viruses (HIV–2) before a clearer picture can emerge [1].

HIV AND TRANSMISSION

Despite the inexorable spread of HIV infection and AIDS world-wide the three main routes of transmission described initially remain the only ones demonstrated to be important. The reason for a comprehensive section on transmission and infection control is that HIV and AIDS is the victim of much discrimination and prejudice based largely on ignorance. We aim to present the facts in a way which is as dispassionate and objective as possible based on recommendations, guidelines and standard clinical practice. This is subject to revision and modification, however the fundamental principles are as follows [2,3].

Table 2.1 Known routes of transmission

Inoculation of blood
- Inoculation of infected blood and blood products.
- Needle sharing among drug misusers.
- Injection with unsterile needles.

Sexual
- Men who have sex with men (homosexual).
- Men who have sex with women, women who have sex with men (heterosexual).

Perinatal
- Inter-uterine transmission from mother to foetus.
- Peripartum, i.e. breast feeding.

Routes investigated and *not* shown to be involved in transmission:
- Close personal contact.
- Household contact.
- Transmission from health care workers unless other risk factors exist.
- Transmission through insect bites.

INFECTION CONTROL

While this section focuses on HIV infection, other associated infections may be more important, as a result of a greater potential for spread. This refers mainly to hepatitis B which is associated with similar client-groups (gay men, drug misusers). The guidelines below are comprehensive and include precautions for hepatitis B as well as HIV infection [3]. There is good evidence that so long as these guidelines are followed the risk to health care workers is very low. Social contacts are clearly at no greater risk [4].

General hygiene procedures should underpin any strategy to

prevent the transmission of infection, irrespective of the human immune deficiency virus. This is even more relevant for those with chronic HIV infection. Such patients with immune impairment are at special risk of acquiring infections and hygiene measures are an important component of care. There are a number of ways the body ensures infections are kept at bay including a complex immune system and the production of antibodies. One of the most practical and important of these is an intact skin which is an extremely effective barrier to infectious diseases. One part of the strategy is to maximize this natural barrier and prevent accidental or unforeseen breaches.

Infection control measures are designed to prevent entry of virus into human body; dispose of and disinfect bodily secretions and excretions, and dispose of and disinfect contaminated material.

Washing hands and using gloves

Hand-washing is one of the most basic of procedures which is of prime importance and should not be overlooked or forgotten.

It should be done properly with soap and hot water before and after contact with contaminated material; before and following preparation of food, and also before and after eating food. This should also occur after contact with each client.

Gloves are required when direct contact will occur between body fluids and the body. Should the contact person have open skin lesions (for example, due to eczema or psoriasis) then this type of work should be avoided. Gloves are not necessary during general, casual contact, for example, if assisting with feeding so long as the skin is intact.

Body fluids and soiling

Where soiling occurs, cleaning ought to occur in two stages: first, hot, soapy water should be used to remove any excretions, and then the area or clothes should be disinfected. Optimal disinfection should utilize sodium hypochlorite solution (1 part household bleach: 10 parts of hot water) which can be used on or in toilets, floors and other surfaces. *Do not use bleach on skin. Bleach can discolour materials like carpets and furnishings.* Note that when using disinfectants, good ventilation of the area is necessary as potentially dangerous gases can be released.

Bedpans and commodes may need regular cleaning especially if incontinence is present or signs of infections persist. Where soiling occurs regularly, carers/relatives/care assistants should wear disposable gowns to protect damage to clothes. Ordinary clothes can be washed in the ordinary home setting provided the machine is set for a 'hot wash', sometimes bleach can be used, especially if soiling has occurred. Disposables such as gloves and paper towels should be placed in a plastic bag, tied up and preferably bagged again prior to discarding.

Sharps

The one major risk to care givers is transmission through a needle stick injury. Overall the risk is still very small and the following practice points should minimize any risk if they are adhered to:

- Do not re-sheath needles.
- Needles and other 'sharps' should be placed, immediately, into a special puncture-resistant container (**sharps-bin**) following the recommended procedure.
- Portable sharps-bins are available for home use. Do not overfill these containers or accidents will occur.
- Last, but not least, take your time. Accidents occur when the care giver is in a hurry and all safety procedures are not followed. It is better to be late and safe than to take unnecessary risks.

Disposal

Local regulations will determine how soiled materials are finally removed and incinerated. The following is a summary:

- Contaminated material for disposal should be placed in heavy-duty plastic bags.
- All sharps, needles and other disposable surgical equipment should be placed in sharps-bins and incinerated.
- Linen which is soiled with body fluids including blood, should be double bagged in heavy-duty plastic bags and collected by properly trained personnel.

- Local policy will determine how instruments are to be cleaned, disinfected and sterilized, i.e. speculae, proctoscopes, etc.

While such precautions are necessary for obvious reasons, the manner in which this aspect of care is delivered will provide a telling insight into overall care. Safety, sensitivity and confidentiality should be the aims of this service.

Table 2.2 Summary of hygiene guidelines

Routine attention to hygiene is satisfactory and the following guidelines may be useful.

- Where blood or other body fluids are spilt, bleach should be used for cleaning (diluted 1:10 with water) and gloves used. If in contact with the skin use only soap and hot water. Do not use bleach on skin.
- Cuts and grazes need only a waterproof dressing until healing with scab formation occurs.
- Where soiling of clothes/sheets has occurred, ordinary machine-washing will suffice provided a 'hot cycle' is used. Gloves ought to be used in handling soiled articles.
- Care is needed with sharps which could carry body fluids, the minimum time sharps are exposed the less likelihood of an accident. Always place sharps in a puncture resistant container ('sharps-bin') immediately after the procedure.
- Razors and toothbrushes should not be shared.
- Crockery, utensils and places should be washed in hot water and detergent as normal.

THE NATURAL HISTORY OF HIV

The relative recent identification of the human immune deficiency virus and its long latency period has meant that many details of its natural history have yet to be clarified and this will continue to be the case for the foreseeable future. However, a wide variation of clinical manifestations is evident from the experience of the first ten years.

The first clear manifestation of the virus is the **seroconversion** illness, but this does not affect all and it may well go unrecognized. It is extremely difficult to differentiate it from many other acute viral infections, the commonest of which include influenza or the common cold. These viruses result in a rapid onset illness: fever, enlarged glands, sore throat, aching muscles and perhaps a rash. In HIV, where this illness occurs (called a glandular fever-type illness) there is usually complete resolution within two or three weeks. In many cases there may be no symptoms whatsoever and a person may seroconvert without any knowledge.

This process, whether associated with a self-limiting illness or not, is called seroconversion and results in the production of antibodies by the body. Antibodies are the body's important cellular defence mechanism against germs, microbes and other unwanted organisms. In the case of HIV infection, these antibodies will confirm that infection with HIV has occurred, though the presence of antibodies within the blood stream may not occur for at least three months.

The period from infection to detectable antibody production is called the *window period* because the blood tests will not reliably confirm or deny the presence of HIV. This is why for some, tests are repeated at three and six-month intervals, in order to verify the result. What happens after seroconversion is the subject of much debate, though there is usually a quiet or latent phase, often for years, where the individual remains trouble-free, enjoying a good quality of life and suffering no symptoms. During this period the individual is still potentially infectious, hence the need for all-round education on safe sex and not sharing dirty needles [5].

Persistent generalized lymphadenopathy (PGL)

The name of this condition describes the syndrome otherwise known as PGL. In essence it represents enlargement of lymph nodes (*lymphadenopathy*) throughout the body (generalized) and which do so over a period of time, initially for longer than three weeks (persistent).

PGL has a technical definition, but there is little more to this condition except that other causes need to be excluded before a diagnosis can be made. For example other infections or tumours, completely unrelated to HIV may be a cause. Simple explanations of why the various lymph node groups react in such a way is not available though closer examination does show 'marked inflammation' and this may represent activity within the immune system of the body.

The syndrome can be associated with constitutional symptoms such as malaise, lethargy and night sweats though overall it has no prognostic value in HIV disease progression. In summary PGL is a diffuse condition representing probably an early phase in the continuum of chronic HIV infection.

AIDS-related complex (ARC)

This now outdated term implied symptomatic disease and was originally used to define individuals with a number of symptoms and signs which were thought to be directly due to chronic HIV infection. Once again, technically certain criteria were used to define whether an individual was within the ARC category or not, though these terms were always arbitrary. The term signified the onset of symptoms and certain conditions associated with chronic HIV infection. Specific infections, although initially trivial can reflect a profound deficiency in the function of the immune system. An example of this includes thrush or candida. 'Symptomatic HIV infection' is now the accepted term for this stage of the condition.

Acquired immune deficiency syndrome (AIDS)

AIDS is the acronym for the Acquired Immune Deficiency Syndrome and represents the most serious manifestation of chronic HIV infection implying severe impairment of the cellular immune system. The poorly functioning immune system therefore leaves the body vulnerable to a large number of infections sometimes called *opportunistic infections*. This group of infections have previously only been prevalent in individuals with severe illness, e.g., those who have undergone renal transplantations.

Another characteristic of AIDS is the high incidence of tumours which can proliferate against this background of a poorly functioning immunity. Certain tumours like non-Hodgkin's type lymphoma are becoming a common complication in individuals with AIDS.

Neurological conditions are also a feature of AIDS and can range from single nerve palsies making little difference to a patient to a debilitating paraparesis restricting function, reducing mobility and severely affecting qualify of life (case history, Chapter 8).

In summary, individuals with AIDS have the most seriously impaired immune systems so allowing infections and cancers to proliferate. While this is so, many with AIDS function well despite their condition and continue to work and enjoy life, though activities may be constrained. These so-called 'long-term survivors' (greater than five years) are commonplace, though why some individuals remain well for so long while others progress rapidly to ill health and advanced disease is unknown.

Table 2.3 Synopsis of common conditions in patients with HIV and AIDS

The following principles act as rules of thumb when treating infections within an HIV compromised patient [6].

- Fungal, parasitic and viral infections are rarely curable, the aim of management is to control these conditions and therefore long-term therapies for prevention may be necessary.
- The majority of infections result from endogenous organisms which have infected the host months or years previously and therefore do not pose a threat to other people. There are exceptions to this, the main ones being tuberculosis (TB) and salmonella.
- Infections will be multiple and therefore a failure to respond to treatment may indicate other infections rather than a failure of initial therapy.
- Frequency of infections is dependent on local geography and environment, i.e., individuals who travel to exotic places often need to be screened for unusual or exotic infections if symptoms and signs suggest.
- Certain bacterial infections are now recognized as being HIV-associated due to extended damage to the immune system.
- Infection due to the compromised immune system may often be severe with multiple sites affected and physical states affected markedly.

A SURVEY OF HIV-RELATED SYMPTOMS AND DISEASES

Table 2.4 Checklist in HIV infection [7]

General constitutional risk
Behaviour
Weight loss
Sweats/night sweats
Well-being

Skin
Dryness
Seborrhoeic dermatitis
Folliculitis
Herpes simplex/zoster

Mouth
Gingivitis
Oral candida
Leukoplakia
Kaposi's sarcoma

Gastrointestinal
Dysphagia
Diarrhoea
Abdominal pain
Perianal disease

The skin

Skin conditions are easily visible and thus are described first. A deteriorating skin condition is often disproportionately disabling and patients may appear distressed and anxious on account of seemingly small and harmless looking lesions.

Dry skin

A common complaint easily recognized but often helped by moisturizing oils and other emollients.

Seborrhoeic dermatitis

A characteristic rash which appears over the forehead, nose and across the cheeks of the face. It can also appear on the trunk and the upper portion of the back where it is usually itchy, sometimes scaly and often red. Treatment usually consists of ointments and creams though emollients do help.

Psoriasis

This is now thought to be specially HIV-related and may occur for the first time in individuals with HIV infection. Treatment consists of emollients and coal tar preparations for maintenance though specialist help is often required where the condition is resistant to treatment.

Molluscum contagiosum

This is a common problem for those with immune deficiency, presenting as small umbilicated papules over face, neck and forehead. Local treatment is usually sufficient though large numbers can occur, especially where immunity is severely affected (Fig. 2.1).

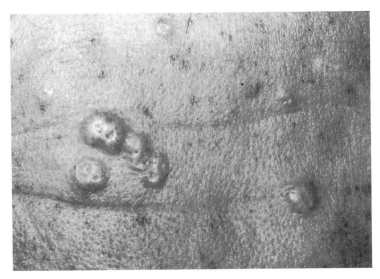

Figure 2.1 Molluscum contagiosum seen on skin of patient with AIDS.

Herpes simplex

Cold sores (types 1 and 2 herpes) are common HIV complaints and affect mouth and genitalia as well as perianal area. Thankfully it is now amenable to therapy and maintenance therapy may be necessary to prevent recurrences. The onset of herpes is a fairly sensitive clinical indicator of immune function though other precipitating factors exist.

Herpes zoster

This is otherwise known as 'shingles' and due to herpes zoster. Shingles arises from a previous episode of herpes zoster most usually known as 'chicken pox' in children – the recurrence is due to an impaired immune system. It usually presents as a nasty sore, red rash covering a dermatome. This can affect the eyes and in these cases specialist advice is needed to prevent blindness.

Kaposi's sarcoma (KS)

In Western countries the second commonest diagnosis conferring on an individual a diagnosis of AIDS [5]. Although now commonly associated with HIV infection, Kaposi's sarcoma was originally described over 100 years ago in Eastern Europe.

Latterly it was found to be more common in certain African countries (Zaire, Kenya, Uganda) where it can constitute up to 10% of all malignancies, mainly in the male population.

KS is a tumour of the cells lining the blood vessels (endothelial cells). These tumours are usually multiple and locally invasive. When present they are flat or raised, painless, purple or dark red spots and sometimes surrounded by bruising (Fig. 2.2). The lesions are often found in prominent areas like the face, forehead and around the eyes. Other areas include the mucous membranes (mouth, penis). Internal KS affecting the gastrointestinal tract or the lungs can be problematic and usually indicates a poorer prognosis.

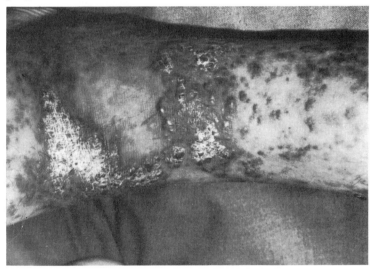

Figure 2.2 Extensive Kaposi's sarcoma on leg of male patient with AIDS.

Treatment of KS is very much dependent on the severity of symptoms. This may range from no treatment for painless skin KS to systemic chemotherapy for life-threatening 'internal' KS. Unsightly or particularly prominent lesions on the face or torso can fade and flatten following radiotherapy which has been used to good effect [8].

Respiratory system

Sinusitis

This is fairly common in individuals with chronic HIV infection. The range of microbes is similar to those in non-infected individuals and usually a course of broad spectrum antibiotics will suffice.

Pneumonia

The features of bacterial pneumonia in individuals with HIV infection are no different from those described in the non-immunocompromised person. Factors such as smoking are important in increasing susceptibility to chest infections and pneumonia. Broad spectrum antibiotics can be used to good effect.

The atypical pneumonias are the ones which receive most notoriety in the field of HIV infection and AIDS, especially the one caused by pneumocystis carinii (PCP). PCP is an infection which can present acutely with signs of pneumonia (shortness of breath, dry cough and fever) or in contrast, can occur insidiously with malaise, flu-type symptoms and a non-specific cough.

PCP is significant because, following confirmation, the patient usually receives an AIDS diagnosis, although the pneumonia is treatable. In the West half of all patients with AIDS have such a diagnosis conferred on them following an episode of PCP [5].

Treatment consists of intravenous antibiotic therapy usually for two weeks though intolerance and side effects of medication, including rashes, can be severe. Milder cases may only necessitate a one-week course of intravenous therapy followed by oral treatment, though close monitoring is necessary.

The role of preventive therapy (prophylactic treatment) is also crucial and will influence the presentation of disease. A number of regimes are in use and this aspect of care has undoubtedly increased survival for those with chronic HIV infection.

Cytomegalovirus (CMV)

Cytomegalovirus is a virus related to the herpes type virus which is a major cause of morbidity in immunocompromised hosts. CMV pneumonia is clinically indistinguishable from PCP. Treatment is again intravenous and usually the duration is two weeks.

Kaposi's sarcoma (KS)

Spread of KS to the lung can present as a pneumonia and a diagnosis is usually made following a bronchoscopy. When widespread throughout the chest, the symptoms include cough, shortness of breath and haemoptysis (coughing blood). Although urgent treatments can improve quality of life, prognosis is very poor.

Mycobacteria

Overall infection with these species of mycobacteria has been found to affect approximately 25% of individuals with AIDS at some stage in their illness.

Mycobacteria tuberculosis (TB) was once extremely common and probably the major cause of death 100 years ago. Due to the major improvements in health, including the environment (adequate housing, clean water and sewage disposal) tuberculosis had declined in prevalence, that is, until recently. However, new evidence suggests that small groups of individuals are becoming increasingly susceptible to TB, including immigrants and people who live in poor socio-economic conditions, e.g., the homeless and drug misusers.

Treatment usually consists of a 9–12 month treatment of triple antibiotic therapy. Once diagnosed, procedures to prevent transmission are necessary since droplet infection is common. However following treatment for 1–2 weeks (in-patient if necessary) individuals may resume normal contact, though this would be dependent on the severity of the illness and the response to treatment. This type of precaution is common for those with or without HIV infection.

Other forms of mycobacteria called MAI (Mycobacteria avium intracellulare or Mycobacteria xenopii) are found in those with HIV infection. These organisms are often found in patients with advanced disease and their exact role is undefined. MAI infection does not pose a risk to others in social contact, and there are no special precautionary measures which need to be established.

Gastrointestinal system

Apthous ulcers

Mucocutaneous herpes and other organisms can affect the mouth in those with HIV disease. Depending on the degree of immuno-compromise it may be difficult to treat and supportive measures may prove to be very important. These include local, topical treatments, steroids and antibiotics as well as anti-viral therapies.

Hairy oral leukoplakia

These are certain lesions within the mouth which are highly characteristic of HIV infection and are present on the sides of the tongue. These are classically painless (though can be painful) and form white, striated patches which do not scrape off. Although they may look benign, these lesions do indicate some progression with chronic HIV infection. It is thought to be due to the Epstein Barr virus, the same organism which causes glandular fever.

Candidiasis, thrush, monilia

All the names are synonymous. Thrush or candida is a ubiquitous fungus which is a profound indicator of an individual's immunity. It is known to affect many parts of the body and is associated with diabetes, steroid therapy or broad spectrum antibiotics. These factors render a person susceptible to candida and it is commonly found in the mouth or other mucous membranes. Women are often affected intermittently with vaginal candida which can be sexually transmitted and can be difficult to eradicate (Fig. 2.3).

With advancing disease, multiple opportunistic infections and widespread antibiotics, thrush is more difficult to control. Here combination treatments can be tried or intravenous therapy for short periods. Also, pulsed or intermittent treatment regimes can be used which hopefully prevents resistance.

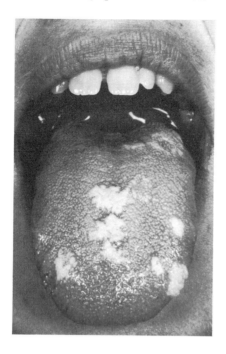

Figure 2.3 Oral thrush (candida) in patient with chronic HIV infection.

Diarrhoea

Diarrhoea is one of the most common symptoms of gastrointestinal disturbance and is usually due to underlying infection. It can also be the most distressing of symptoms, especially if severity renders the individual debilitated and incontinent which is not all that infrequent.

The commonest infections will be highlighted, though it is important to stress that symptoms may result from HIV alone irrespective of underlying or superadded infections. Investigations for this condition include stool samples, in-patient monitoring and endoscopy/colonoscopy as well as barium studies.

Salmonella

Salmonella is one of the few organisms which constitute a special risk for a patient with HIV infection since it is difficult to eradicate and thus may be transmitted to others. It is treated aggressively, usually on an in-patient basis, where special precautions need to be taken to prevent spread (single room, isolation, barrier nursing). If mild, it can be treated on an out-patient basis.

Cryptosporidia/microsporidia

Probably the commonest cause of diarrhoea in someone with AIDS, the diagnosis is made by isolation of this protozoa within the stool or bowel wall on at least two occasions. Cryptosporidiosis is an AIDS-defining condition and very difficult to treat. Symptoms are commonly loose, watery diarrhoea with flatulence, profound urgency often resulting in incontinence.

Spread of cryptosporidium to the biliary system can cause great pain and is difficult to treat except with palliative measures. A number of antibiotics have been tried with little sustained benefit.

Measures to try and reduce diarrhoea are an important objective of care, these include loperamide/codeine/morphine preparations. Some thought needs to be given to access to the toilet and incontinence pads if this continues.

The natural course of the infection is one which fluctuates, and paradoxically periods of constipation may occur especially if potent anti-diarrhoeals are used (opiates or morphine-type mixtures).

Cryptosporidial outbreaks have occurred in drinking water, generating understandable alarm. The non-immunocompromised population will not usually be affected by these outbreaks.

Cytomegalovirus (CMV) infection

These viruses are again extremely common and represent a flu-type illness in those who are non-immunocompromised. However, in HIV infection, chronic relapsing CMV may be characteristic and within the gastrointestinal system may cause diarrhoea, abdominal pain, incontinence, abdominal distension and fever as well as malaise and general ill-health.

Abdominal tenderness is often characteristic and treatment is confined to intravenous preparations usually for 2–3 weeks per episode. Usually prophylaxis is not required, though this is dependent on severity and frequency of episodes. Another condition characteristic of CMV disease is ulceration, usually oesophageal which may respond well to treatment.

Mycobacterium avium intracellulare infection (MAI)

In advanced disease Mycobacterium avium intracellulare (MAI) may be isolated within the gut where it can cause diarrhoea and other constitutional symptoms. There is little evidence to suggest treatments will increase longevity though empirical treatment may reduce symptoms and enhance quality of life. As previously discussed, their exact role is undefined, although treatment is usually associated with improvement of some symptoms.

HIV

Human immune deficiency virus may directly affect cells of the gastrointestinal tract causing inflammation, with diarrhoea and pain. Chronic symptoms may result in malabsorption and may contribute to the weight loss seen so often in individuals with chronic HIV infection (Chapter 5). Diagnosis is usually dependent on excluding other treatable infections.

Nervous system

The various neurological manifestations of chronic HIV infections and AIDS are now recognized to be multiple, often complex and all too often not remediable. The added dimension within this subgroup is the relationship between organic disease and the psychological response to the various conditions. When there has been a recent onset of psychological symptoms organic disease needs to be excluded before a full psychiatric evaluation can take place.

Toxoplasmosis

This is an infection caused by a protozoa. A failing immune system will result in active infection, usually from latent organisms. Blood testing often shows that a substantial proportion of the population have previously been infected, usually when very young.

An acute presentation may include constitutional symptoms (fever, headache, vomiting, fits) as well as motor or sensory symptoms. Acute symptoms affecting speech with ataxia (co-ordination problems) may also indicate infection. Diagnosis usually follows a Computerized tomography (CT) or Magnetic Resonance Imaging (MRI) scan (Fig. 2.4). Treatment consists of anti-toxoplasma therapy, but needs to be continued for a prolonged period, often with prophylactic therapies.

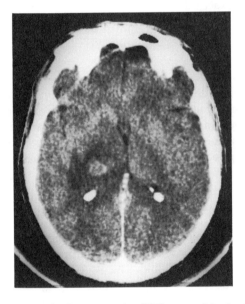

Figure 2.4 Computerized tomography (CT) scan of brain showing multiple toxoplasma abscesses in patient with AIDS.

Cryptococcus neoformans

This fungal infection which is the commonest cause of meningitis usually presents with headache, fever, photophobia, neck stiffness or rigidity. The presentation may however be more indolent and gradual, and hence symptoms may last 2–4 weeks before diagnosis. The definitive investigation is a lumbar puncture and a cerebrospinal (CSF) sample can be analysed for infection with cryptococcus. Anti-fungal therapy is usually intravenous. Prophylactic therapy is mandatory, to prevent recurrence.

Cytomegalovirus (CMV)

This viral infection is extremely common and a significant proportion of individuals have had evidence of past infection.

However in certain groups like drug misusers, kidney transplant patients and also gay men, up to 95% of individuals have had previous infection. In those with immune deficiency, infection can be severe and generalized affecting, either singularly or in combination, the gastrointestinal tract respiratory system, and nervous system. Treatment needs to be aggressive and therefore intravenous, though oral medications are being developed.

The two major neurological problems associated with cytomegalovirus are encephalitis and retinitis. CMV encephalitis presents with confusion, fever and vomiting; fairly rapid deterioration is not uncommon. CMV retinitis presents with deteriorating vision, sudden onset of 'floaters' within the eye (black dots which appear to float across the eye) or partial loss of vision. These symptoms all necessitate an urgent specialist opinion. Because therapy may be prolonged and since treatment is intravenous, long-term access to veins is necessary and consequently this regime is relatively invasive. For those individuals with CMV retinitis, the aim of therapy is to control infection and prevent further deterioration; sometimes there is limited improvement in visual acuity.

Progressive multifocal leucoencephalopathy

This rather ostentatiously named condition describes well its manifestations: 'multifocal' – multiple; 'leuco' – affecting the white matter; 'encephalopathy' – resulting in deteriorating brain function, and 'progressive' meaning prognosis is poor. It is thought to result from a previously latent virus, and presumably this is activated at times of immune impairment.

AIDS-related dementia

Dementia simply denotes a global impairment of function including personality changes, memory loss, social skills and concentration. AIDS-related dementia means that these changes are directly due to HIV infection in the absence of other opportunistic infections. Antiretroviral therapies have demonstrated some benefit though overall prognosis is poor.

This condition represents a major challenge for all health care workers as well as for partners, families and carers of those affected. The physical, psychological and social manifestations of this condition can be immense and the full array of services within a community may need mobilizing if the person is to remain at home (Chapter 8).

REFERENCES

1. Adler, M.W. (ed.) *ABC of AIDS*, BMA Publications, London, 1984.
2. Miller, D., Green, J. and Weber, J. *The management of AIDS patients*, Macmillan Press, Basingstoke, UK, 1986.
3. BMA (Professional Division) *A Code of Practice for Sterilisation of Instruments and control of infection*, British Medical Association, London, 1989.
4. Morgan, D. (1990) AIDS, HIV and Occupational Health. The AIDS Letter, **20**, Royal Society of Medicine, London.
5. Cohen, P.T., Sande, M.A. and Volberding, P.A. (eds.) *The AIDS Knowledge Base*, The Medical Publishing Group, Waltham, Massachusetts, 1990.
6. Glat, A., Chirgwin, K. and Landesman, S. (1988) Treatment of Infections associated with Human Immunodeficiency Virus. *New England Journal of Medicine*, **318**, 1439–1448.
7. BMA Foundation for AIDS. *The management of HIV infection in Primary care*, British Medical Association Foundation for AIDS, London, 1990.
8. Youle, M.C., *et al. AIDS: Therapeutics in HIV Disease*, Churchill Livingstone, Edinburgh, 1988.

3

The role of the occupational therapist

Louise Cusack

'There is always a new challenge. You look for solutions that give as much independence as possible.'

S. Gore, *District Occupational Therapy*,
Health Services Careers Leaflet 18,
London, March 1990 [1].

Occupational therapists work with people who have a physical and/or mental illness or handicap or a severe injury, enabling them to overcome the effects of their disability and adjust to everyday living. They teach patients ways of building up physical and psychological strength, counselling them on how to cope with temporary or permanent disability, and the varied demands of daily life [2].

The World Federation of Occupational Therapy defines occupational therapy as 'the treatment of physical and psychiatric conditions through specific activities in order to help people reach their maximum level of function and independence in all aspects of daily life' [3]. Bearing in mind it is a relatively new and still developing profession and one of the fastest growing paramedical professions, the occupational therapist has a fundamental role in the management and care of people with HIV infection and AIDS.

Over the years, occupational therapists have been found in hospital-based settings, providing rehabilitation and treatment for a number of chronic illnesses and a disabled population. Historically they have responded with a biomechanical approach – treatment in terms of strengthening muscles and widening range of movement. However, with the development of new approaches, occupational therapists, working in non-traditional settings, have addressed the challenge of working with people with HIV/AIDS and created a truly holistic approach to care.

The disabilities that result from AIDS (cancer, hemiplegia, adjustment reactions, cognitive disorders, blindness, etc.) do not require a change in occupational therapy intervention approaches.

However, occupational therapists working with people with AIDS may be more effective if they use the 'whole person' concept to address the psychosocial, physical, and environmental factors influencing function [4]. An occupational therapist's holistic training enables patients not only to maintain function and improve independence but they are able to facilitate choices, which are to be made by the patient in all aspects of everyday activity and living.

As such, occupational therapists have a vital and key role within the larger multidisciplinary team. They contribute an important part in the overall care plan and package, that is available to the patient, from early intervention of a newly-diagnosed HIV positive patient to terminal and palliative care of the patient with AIDS.

If the occupational therapist's role is to facilitate and promote maximum function in daily activity and to enable the patient to achieve his personal goals, it is important that a good relationship is developed early on between the patient and the therapist, and that this is maintained, possibly over a period of many years. Obviously the occupational therapist will not be directly in contact at all times, however, the patient is aware of how to contact the occupational therapist at points of need or crisis.

A patient with HIV infection or AIDS may be referred to an occupational therapist at any stage of illness. However it is more likely that the referral will be made when a patient has presented a symptomatic disease. All information given by the patient must be respected and remain confidential throughout all stages of the treatment programme.

It is also important to clarify at the point of referral, which other team members are, or may be, involved in the patients care. This can also be discussed with the patient on the initial assessment. The initial assessment will primarily be an interview, in order to gather information, and identify areas of further need and assessment, and areas of treatment and interaction.

GENERAL PRINCIPLES OF TREATMENT

Patient autonomy

This is fundamental in the care of the patient and must be upheld throughout the course of treatment. So often a patient loses autonomy within the hospital system. Patient autonomy should allow the person to make choices and take responsibility for himself and his progress. A safe and non-judgmental environment must be created to enable the person to function to their optimum level.

Joint planning

The occupational therapist and the patient should plan together to identify treatment goals. This is essential in the overall care of a patient as it creates a greater understanding of a particular approach used, and it enables decision-making to be shared.

Communication

Communication is of paramount importance. To ensure communication is successful and effective, the use of language and its style must be familiar to the patient and the use of special terminology and jargon avoided at all costs, particularly when addressing more difficult and sensitive issues.

Multidisciplinary team work

The occupational therapist will work within a large multidisciplinary team, both within and outside the hospital environment, and will need to liaise with a variety of different disciplines depending on the nature of the problem.

Within the hospital

- Doctors
- Nurses
- Dieticians
- Physiotherapists
- Social workers
- Chaplains
- Health education workers
- Chiropodists
- Clinical psychologists
- Psychiatrists
- Health advisers

Outside the hospital

- Community occupational therapists
- Social workers
- Home helps
- Home carers

- General practitioners
- Specialist nurses
- District nurses
- Volunteers

INTERVENTION

Occupational therapy intervention may take place in individual sessions, or, in contrast, within a group setting. Each method of intervention will depend on the nature of the treatment. Intervention must be tailored to the individual needs of the patient, as he may enter treatment at any stage of disease. However, individual treatment usually takes on the form of specific tasks and goals, whereas groupwork may offer more generalized treatment aims.

Groupwork

A closed group

A 'closed group' is one where the members are selected or choose to be in the group, and those same members meet for a predetermined number of sessions. New members are not allowed to enter and present members are not allowed to leave. Usually the group will make contracts; these may lead to fairly intense work. An example of such a group would be an encounter group.

A slow open group

A 'slow open group' is one where new members join and old members leave; members being selected by themselves. The group will meet regularly and again is supportive in nature. An example of such a group would be a creative art group.

Individual intervention treatment

Below are outlined the areas of intervention an occupational therapist may become involved in. It is not prescriptive but is given to highlight areas in which the therapist works.

Table 3.1 Areas of intervention involving the occupational therapist

Early intervention
• Emotional support
• Personal activities of daily living and self-care
• Home management
• General mobility
• Energy conservation
• Stress management and relaxation techniques
• Employment and leisure

Late intervention
All of the above and
• Disability equipment
• Housing and home assessment
• Leisure and social activities
• Groupwork and creative self-expression

Loss of independence in many areas may be affected for a variety of different reasons and intervention must therefore take into account the underlying cause. For example:

• Neurological problems such as peripheral neuropathy or hemiplegia.
• Psychological difficulties, including a lack of motivation or depression.
• Lethargy and weakness caused for example by tuberculosis (TB) or anaemia.
• Memory loss as in HIV encephalopathy or progressive multifocal leucoencephalopathy (PML) [5].
• Visual impairment or loss of sight by cytomegalovirus.

EMOTIONAL SUPPORT AND COUNSELLING

The occupational therapist must be aware of the patient's psychological state throughout involvement. Each patient's needs will be very different, for example, the patient who has lost his sight as a result of cytomegalovirus will not only have to cope with the physical loss but also the psychological impact. A patient may be involved with other professionals and have a supportive network of friends, therefore it is important for the patient to maintain contact with them. However, while the therapist is in contact with the patient, she may have to support the patient, particularly around issues with loss and disability. The therapist is often the best person to assist the patient in working through these issues.

The occupational therapist will need to support the patient and/ or carers in assessing future needs. Decision-making will require great sensitivity and trust as various options for resettlement and care are considered. At times, this will be difficult for the patient, so the therapist must be able to explore the options and support any decisions made. Both emotional and physical support will be needed during the later stages of disease, particularly if the patient chooses to be cared for at home.

Much time must be spent with carers as fears and anxiety usually present with physical difficulties. The therapist may find themselves closely involved with the partner or family. It will be important to recognize their needs, and offer appropriate support, e.g., practical help, information and resources (Table 3.2) [6].

Table 3.2 Carers' needs

---
1. Recognition of their contribution and of their own needs as individuals in their own right.
2. Services tailored discussions at the time help is being planned.
3. Services which reflect an awareness of differing sexual orientations and racial, cultural and religious backgrounds and values, equally accessible to carers of every race and ethnic origin.
4. Opportunities for a break, both for short spells (an afternoon) and for longer periods (a week or more), to relax and have time to themselves.
5. Practical help to lighten the tasks of caring, including domestic help, home adaptations, incontinence services and help with transport.
6. Someone to talk to about their own emotional needs, at the outset of caring, while they are caring, and when the caring task is over.
7. Information about available benefits and services as well as how to cope with the particular condition of the individual cared for.
8. An income which covers the costs of caring and which does not preclude carers taking employment or sharing care with other people.
9. Opportunities to explore alternatives to family care, both for immediate and long-term future.
10. Services designed through consultation with carers, at all levels of policy planning.

DAILY LIVING AND SELF-CARE

Personal activities of daily living and self-care include activities such as personal hygiene, grooming, bathing and dressing. Those tasks may be extremely tiring and take much effort. It is important to try and establish routines and to allow adequate time, as rushing may cause more stress than necessary.

Bathing and toiletting

Taking a bath may be a very therapeutic, relaxing and enjoyable task; paradoxically, it may also be very tiring and exhausting. It may be advisable to take a bath at the end of a day when rest can be taken immediately afterwards. The bath water must not be too hot as this in itself may prove overwhelming. If oils are used in the bath, again, caution must be given and possibly a non-slip bath mat used. Place the toilet lid down or have a small stool that can be used to sit on while undressing and dressing, and when towelling down.

Grab rails and the use of a padded bath board and padded bath seat may facilitate independence, however if a soak is preferred these will prove cumbersome. Therefore bathing with a padded bath cushion and some assistance may prove necessary (Figs. 3.1

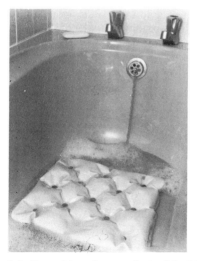

Figure 3.1 Padded bath cushion for comfort of bathing. (Photograph -courtesy of Keep Able Ltd, Wellingborough, Northants.)

and 3.2). If a shower is preferred then again a non-slip shower mat, grab rails and a perching stool may facilitate a safe shower (Fig. 3.3). On the toilet, a padded or raised toilet seat with grab rails, may be fitted for comfort.

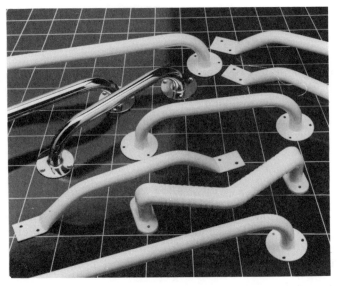

Figure 3.2 Selection of grab rails. (Photograph courtesy of Keep Able Ltd, Wellingborough, Northants.)

Any equipment placed in the bathroom must be safe and functional. It must be discussed with the patient as they may be sharing their bathroom with others. There may be a need to explain to a carer how the equipment is fitted and used in order to safeguard against accidents. In the later stages of intervention a hoist may be necessary. This must be assessed accurately before it is supplied.

Home management

Home management is the ability to take an active role in the smooth running of the home, i.e. cleaning, shopping and laundry. This role may vary in different states of health and disease, and it is important to involve the patient even as a 'back seat driver' e.g. assistance in meal planning, making shopping lists.

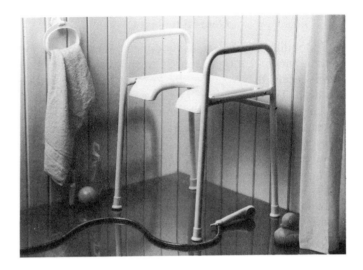

Figure 3.3 Shower stool. (Photograph courtesy of Keep Able Ltd, Wellingborough, Northants.)

Modern appliances such as washing machines, tumble dryers, fridge/freezers and microwaves will be essential. Other electrical appliances such as an electric tin opener and food processor not only will be useful but will enable the patient to conserve personal strength, and stay independent for longer.

Household tasks may need to be reduced to just light duties, whilst the heavier tasks such as cleaning and ironing are left to willing helpers. If practical help is available at home, this will be beneficial to allow the patient time and energy to carry out the activities he wishes to do. Help at home may vary from private cleaning arrangements to 'Homehelp' provided by the Department of Social Services. Charitable agencies may offer volunteers to assist in cooking, shopping and laundry, etc.

The patient may need some time to adjust to, and accept the reality of, accepting strangers into the home and allowing them to take on household responsibilities. However once trust can be placed with the 'help', the advantages far outweigh the disadvantages.

General mobility

General mobility may be relatively difficult early on in HIV disease due to anaemia, fatigue, muscle-wasting and lethargy; advice and intervention may together be given with advice on energy conservation. The emphasis will be on general mobility for activities of daily living, to enable the individual to maintain independence and manage short distances without experiencing breathlessness or fatigue.

For walking sticks or crutches, a joint assessment with a physiotherapist is advantageous. The physiotherapist may prescribe treatment and exercise programmes that may be then carried out by the individual, often with the assistance of a carer, at home. Lifting and handling of the patient may need to be demonstrated and practised with the carer/s as it is essential that the patient feels safe, and that carers are confident and also know how to avoid back injury.

Eligibility for benefits available, such as free bus passes or 'parking for the disabled' registration should be investigated, and the benefits applied for when the criteria are met. The occupational therapist must be aware of such benefits in order to advise the individual accurately.

Wheelchair mobility

Towards the end of the disease a wheelchair may be prescribed. The issuing of this particular piece of equipment may raise very specific issues relating to disease, illness, loss of independence, prognosis and death. This is extremely important and must be discussed with the individual.

A wheelchair may be required for occasional indoor use or for outdoors. The assessment for the prescription of a wheelchair should take into consideration the following [7]:

The user

- Height and width
- Weight
- Ability and dexterity
- Attitude towards the wheelchair
- Cognitive ability

The place of use

- In the home
- Outside the home
- Day centres, work

Other transport facilities

- Fitting in a car, bus, etc.

Other carers

- Knowledge in use of the chair
- Assistance to be given

Stability

- Outside environment, i.e. pavement and slopes
- Extra fixtures to chair

Cushions

- Posture
- Seating
- Cost
- Durability
- Care

Energy conservation

Energy conservation is important in all activities of daily life, particularly because people with AIDS are prone to profound weakness and lethargy. In order to help save energy the individual could be advised to:

- Use labour-saving equipment such as electric tin openers,

microwave cookers, perching stools, intercom systems and stair lifts.

- Always sit rather than stand.
- Consider carefully before starting a large task that may be difficult to interrupt or stop altogether.
- Pace himself and take frequent rests during quiet moments of the day.
- Plan his day's activities and reserve his energy for the priorities in his life, for example, time spent with loved ones and leisure activities [8].

Stress management and relaxation techniques

It is natural for anyone to have a physical and/or emotional response to a situation that is actually or imagined to be threatening to their physical or emotional well-being and safety. However, stress occurs when the physical and emotional demands made on an individual exceed their resources to deal with them. When this happens stress reduces the ability to cope with everyday problems. The occupational therapist, with the patient, first needs to identify the situations that cause stress, then recognize the signs and effects of feeling stress and, finally, offer positive methods of overcoming those situations (Table 3.3).

Table 3.3 The effects of stress

- Tension headache, dizziness.
- Insomnia.
- Tight/aching neck or shoulders.
- Eyestrain or blurred vision.
- Different sleeping patterns.
- Disrupted eating patterns.
- Skin complaints.
- Incorrect breathing and palpitations.
- Constant tiredness.
- Feeling tense or edgy.
- Short temperedness or unusual impatience.
- Poor concentration span.

Stress management may take on different forms and it is important to determine which method is most appropriate. Techniques such as 'progressive relaxation', 'autogenic training' or 'imagery' are all techniques which may be used in conjunction with breathing exercises (Table 3.4) [9].

Table 3.4 Relaxation techniques

Progressive relaxation
The person learns to become aware of different muscle groups, and how to systematically tense and relax them in turn.

Autogenic training
The person learns how to become systematically aware of each part of the body – head, hand, wrist, forearm, etc. while imagining each part as heavy and warm.

Imagery
The person learns how to conduct himself or be conducted through an imaginary story, for example, taking a peaceful holiday or flying through the sky.

Obviously, the greatest application for these techniques is in the field of health education and primary care. It is not necessary for an individual to wait until an anxiety problem has developed before benefiting from training.

Disability equipment

At any stage of disease the consultation or direct service may be helpful to patients who need simple assistive devices such as a magnifying glass or book holder; a level indicator to help in the pouring of liquids; a 'pill mill' to assist in the correct dispensing of pills, or a baby alarm to allow the carers to hear the patient with AIDS if in another room. All of these will help patients to maintain functional independence [9].

The assessment and selection of particular pieces of disability equipment must always be done in consultation with the patient and carers if appropriate, and mutually agreed upon. It is important to give choices to the patient and explain the reason why a piece of equipment may be useful; careful consideration must be given in prescribing permanent items of equipment. The occupational therapist could set up a 'load system', thus enabling pieces of equipment to be sent out for assessment and then ordered once assessment time is complete. Table 3.5 is a list of disability equipment that has been proved useful in the maintenance of both personal and domestic activities of daily living.

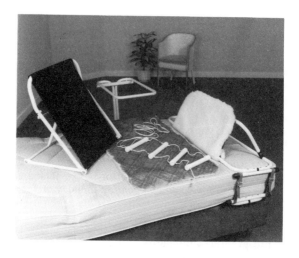

Figure 3.4 Disability equipment used in the bedroom, including a pillow raise, sheepskin and rope ladder. (Photograph courtesy of Keep Able Ltd, Wellingborough, Northants.)

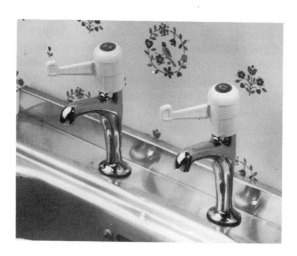

Figure 3.5 Tap turners. (Photograph courtesy of Keep Able Ltd, Wellingborough, Northants.)

Table 3.5 Disability equipment for personal and domestic activities

Personal activities of daily living

Bath seat, bath board, non-slip bath mat, non-slip shower mat, tap turners, grab rails, raised toilet seat, padded toilet seat, and padded perching stool.

Easy reader, 'pill mill', magnifying glass, long-handled shoehorn, Velcro-fastenings on clothes, socket extension (Fig. 3.7).

Raising blocks for the bed, V-shaped pillow, sheepskin, rope ladder, overhead reaching pole, night-light plug, urine bottle with lid (Fig. 3.4).

Domestic activities of daily living

Tap turners and 3 (Figs. 3.5 and 3.6), kettle pourer, electric tin opener, perching stool, level indicator.

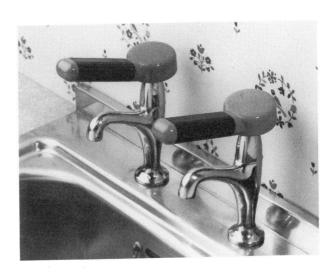

Figure 3.6 Tap turners. (Photograph courtesy of Keep Able Ltd, Wellingborough, Northants.)

Home assessment visit

Throughout the course of a patient's life, he may well only spend about 20% of this time within a health care setting, be that a hospital or hospice, etc. [10]. Therefore it is fundamental that the home provides stability and familiarity.

During a patient's stay in hospital it may be necessary, prior to discharge, for the occupational therapist to carry out a home assessment with the patient, to identify his needs for independent living, particularly after a long period of time in hospital.

Whenever a home assessment visit is carried out, agreement must be sought from the patient, and a full explanation of why the assessment visit is to be carried out. Referral to other agencies and involvement of other team members on the visits may be necessary.

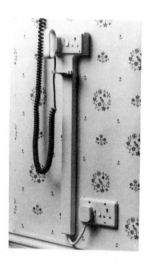

Figure 3.7 A socket raised by an extension. (Photograph courtesy of Keep Able Ltd, Wellingborough, Northants.)

Employment, leisure and social activities

How a patient spends their time following a positive antibody HIV test or an AIDS diagnosis will vary considerably, and depend largely on the nature of the work or activity previous to their diagnosis. There will need to be many considerations based on finance, role, sickness and status when considering the continuing or the termination of employment. Perhaps a change in the working environment or schedule may be sought in order to continue a work role. However, if the patient no longer works, then time may need to be spent looking at his activity wants and how best these may be met, for example, as a volunteer in a related charity. The gains from working or being involved in leisure activities can be considerable, and these activities, if appropriate, should be encouraged.

Often, patients with HIV who are introduced to different organizations find a supportive network, and may feel less need for therapeutic intervention. This is an obvious progression of the therapist's work.

Case History
M.F. was admitted to the ward with sight problems and headaches with an increasing inability to manage at home and work. His right eye had complete visual loss and his left eye had vision but was slightly blurred. He was diagnosed with cytomegalovirus retinitus (CMV). M.F. was daignosed HIV positive in 1985. In 1986 he had non-specific night sweat's and weight loss. On a previous admission to hospital, M.F. had been diagnosed and treated for pneumocystis carinii pneumonia (PCP).

Social history
M.F. lives alone in his privately-owned basement garden flat. Prior to his admission he was working as a computer operator, driving to and from work. He is a keen tennis player and a member of a gay tennis group. He is a popular man with a wide circle of friends, in particular a woman friend at work, but she is unaware of his diagnosis. He has no contact with his family.

Reason for referral to occupational therapy service
Unable to manage at work or home, M.F. required full occupational therapy assessment while in hospital due to recent CMV diagnosis.

Occupational therapy intervention
With close liaison and counselling with the social worker, M.F. decided to retire from work. The occupational therapist's role therefore was to work with M.F. on his sensory, productivity, self-maintenance and leisure skills. It was also important to prevent his social isolation and maintain a safe environment. The intervention included re-orientating himself with his room and the ward environment, feeding himself, maintaining personal hygiene and mobilizing safely around the ward environment. This improvement continued once he had left hospital by slowly regaining familiarity with objects

and furniture at home. As he was no longer able to drive, he needed to familiarize himself with public transport which he did with the help of a 'buddy' from the Terrence Higgins Trust and friends. Eventually, gaining confidence, he started to go to a support group and meet a number of new friends. His friend from work became a key carer and she was supported by home care and voluntary organizations.

Conclusion

With the above action, M.F. was able to continue his life, and be cared for, at home. A support network was developed with the occupational therapist involved on a regular basis to review and evaluate intervention and support the carer.

INTERVENTION IN PALLIATIVE CARE

In recent years modern medicine has become so preoccupied with prevention and cure that the dying patient may be regarded as a failure but we must remember the need of the dying is to be allowed to live.

On the whole, the skills required are the same as in most other areas; however, the therapist needs to feel comfortable and have an ability to tolerate close contact with the dying and with death [11].

Occupational therapy should be based on established relationships, that of patient and family, patient and nurse, patient and multidisciplinary team. Teamwork is essential in providing an overall consistent care package, that is, care given to maintain the patient's dignity, humaneness and quality of life (Table 3.6).

FACING THE CHALLENGE

The occupational therapist ought to be one of the key members within the multidisciplinary team, as they bring with them skills from both a physical as well as a psychological knowledge base. This enables them to focus not only on the acute aspects of HIV infection and AIDS but also the psychosocial and psychological aspects that may present within the spectrum of illness and wellness [12].

Occupational therapy then can enhance a patient's quality of life; the therapist is an important part of the team involved in

Table 3.6 Intervention in palliative care

Life skills
- Personal and home care
- Mobility
- Adaptive equipment

Emotional support
- Relaxation techniques
- Anxiety management
- Groupwork
- Creative self-expression

Social and leisure activities
- Groupwork
- Visits/outings
- New skills taught, for example, art
- Creative skills

Resettlement
- Home assessment
- Home v hospital v hospice
- Community care/multidisciplinary work
- Discharge planning

patient care, and can provide a purpose and sense of fulfilment within the patient's environment.

REFERENCES

1. Gore, S. (March 1990) *District Occupational Therapy*, Health Service Careers Leaflet, HSC18, HMSO.
2. Ibid.
3. World Federation of Occupational Therapists. (May 1989) British Journal of Occupational Therapy, *Occupational Therapy News*, **52**:5.
4. Denton, R. (July 1987) AIDS: Guidelines for Occupational Therapy Intervention, *The American Journal of Occupational Therapy*, **41**, 7.
5. Turner, A., Foster, M., Johnson, S.E. *Occupational Therapy and Physical Dysfunction, Principles, Skills and Practice*, Churchill Livingstone, Edinburgh, 1990, p. 816.
6. *Carers Needs – A 10 Point Plan for Carers* (1989), Published by the Kings Fund and Informal Caring Programme with financial support from Health Education Authority and the Department of Health, England.
7. Turner, *op. cit.*, pp. 280–281.
8. Turner, *op. cit.*, p. 813.
9. Denton, R., *op. cit.*, pp. 427–432.
10. The Second National AIDS Conference, *Care in the Community*, Conference Readings, 28 September 1988–1 October 1988.

11. Kübler-Ross, E. *On Death and Dying*, Tavistock Publications, London, 1970.
12. Pizzi, M. (March 1990) The Transformation of HIV Infection and AIDS in Occupational Therapy: Beginning the Conversation. *The American Journal of Occupational Therapy*, **44**, 3.

4

The role of the physiotherapist

Jenny McClure

INTRODUCTION

People living with HIV and AIDS may require physiotherapy for a wide variety of physical problems. As part of a multidisciplinary team, physiotherapists have much to offer this patient group in the way of advice, treatment and symptom control. Physiotherapy aims to improve the quality of life of a person by reducing or eliminating discomfort and enabling a person to function as well as possible according to their wishes.

These treatment goals should be client-led; although encouragement and explanation of the potential benefits of treatment are important, goals and treatments have to be continually re-evaluated and updated according to changes in the patient's condition or circumstances. Physiotherapists need to work closely with other members of the team as problems related to medical, psychological and social aspects all influence the outcome of physiotherapy treatment.

In this chapter, physiotherapy treatment will be considered in areas of medical speciality and will also include measures that may be initiated in the asymptomatic phase of infection. It should, however, be remembered that sometimes many different symptoms coexist, necessitating adaptation of treatment to meet the patient's needs. Purist methods of treatment may not always be appropriate.

GENERAL HEALTH MEASURES

Exercise

While many patients living with HIV infection wish simply to carry on with their lives as normal, others may wish to become actively involved in 'fighting' the disease from an early stage.

These patients may request advice on suitable exercise regimes. Exercise can be both uplifting and empowering, something positive a person can do for themselves, as opposed to the many treatments in which they are passive recipients.

It is difficult to estimate to what extent exercise will effect the disease process in the long term, although research into the long-term effects of aerobic exercise on HIV positive asymptomatic individuals is currently under way. Several studies indicate that in the short term, aerobic exercise has a positive effect on physical, psychological and immunological parameters in patients with HIV disease, in that it improves general fitness, reduces stress and depression and may even have a positive influence on the immune system [1,2]. It has also been shown that a 6-week progressive resistance exercise regime on a group of patients in the recovery period following an episode of pneumocystis carinii pneumonia (PCP) resulted in improvements in muscle bulk and strength in a six week training programme, compared to a control group who continued to deteriorate in these parameters in the post-acute period [3]. In the absence of long-term studies but in the knowledge that muscle-wasting and general cardiovascular deconditioning are predominant features of this condition, it seems wise to try and prevent these occurring with a combination of aerobic and strengthening exercises.

Prior to commencing an exercise programme, it is useful to consult a dietician to ensure adaptation in nutritional intake to compensate for increased energy expenditure (Chapter 5).

Fitness testing is sometimes appropriate in order to obtain baseline measurements and assess a patient's tolerance to exercise. It should be noted that patients with HIV infection have been shown to exercise to lower workloads than those without HIV infection even when asymptomatic [4,5].

Relaxation

Stress is thought to have a negative effect on the immune system. Techniques that alleviate stress may therefore have benefits other than simply to decrease levels of anxiety. It is valuable to have skills in teaching relaxation techniques, particularly in conditions such as HIV and AIDS where stress is common at all stages. Pain and breathlessness can both be exacerbated by or result in stress. Relaxation may help to alleviate some of these symptoms. There are many different relaxation techniques which will appeal to different patients. As mentioned above, exercise has also been shown to reduce stress and may be a useful adjunct or alternative to other methods of stress reduction (Chapter 3).

Symptomatic HIV-infection and AIDS fatigue

Fatigue is common in HIV infection, it usually fluctuates from day to day and may be profound, causing limitations in the person's ability to function in all but the most sedentary tasks. Fatigue can be a limiting factor in physiotherapy treatment and assessment will have to be made of the relative advantages and disadvantages of additional energy expenditure. If fatigue is a problem then short physiotherapy sessions are indicated and treatment programmes need to be modified accordingly (Chapter 8).

RESPIRATORY COMPLICATIONS

Respiratory complications in patients with chronic HIV infection are common. Physiotherapists may be involved in diagnosis and long-term treatment of such conditions and, in addition, prophylactic therapy.

Pneumocystis Carinii Pneumonia (PCP)

Physiotherapy involvement

Pneumocystis carinii pneumonia (PCP) is the most common and serious respiratory complication in HIV infection and is also AIDS-defining (Chapter 2). The role of the physiotherapist will vary according to the centre in which they work and some of the procedures described here will be carried out by different personnel depending on the treatment centre. Patients themselves can be supervised such that many become adapt at performing their own procedures.

Prophylaxis

See Figs. 4.1–4.4 for some of the methods used to deliver drugs to the patient.

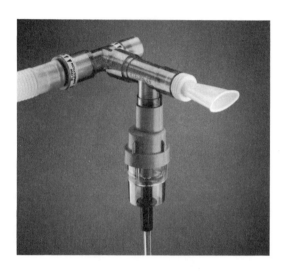

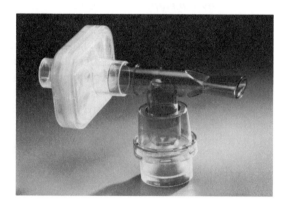

Figure 4.1 Assortment of nebulizers for delivery of pentamidine.

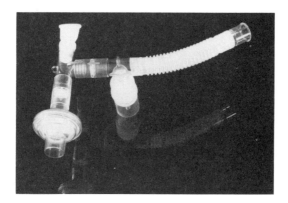

Figure 4.1 Contd.

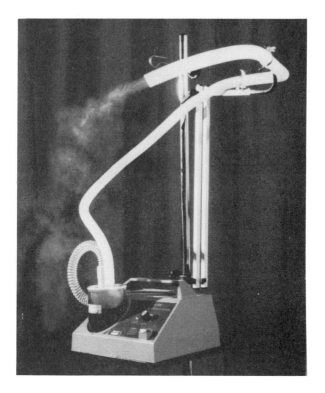

Figure 4.2 Ultrasonic nebulizer for inducing sputum.

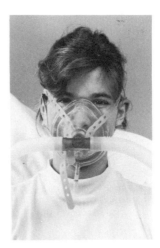

Figure 4.3 The CPAP face mask.

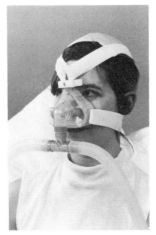

Figure 4.4 The nasal CPAP face mask.

Treatment of PCP

Nebulization of pentamidine

A nebulizer is a small plastic unit driven by a compressor which allows a liquid drug to be 'aerosolized', that is transformed into multiple droplets which can then be inhaled. Nebulization of drugs allows direct delivery of the therapy to the lungs in a form which can be utilized by the lung. The antibiotic pentamidine is a form of anti-PCP therapy. It may be nebulized as primary or secondary prophylaxis for patients and is usually given once or twice a month. The equipment used is of vital importance as it influences the actual delivery of the drug [6]. The appropriate equipment should ensure that the particle size is correct, prevent environmental contamination and maintain acceptability to the patient. If the particle size is too large it will result in deposition of the pentamidine in the upper airways, leading to increased cough and reduced efficacy and compliance. Despite a number of comparative studies on nebulizer equipment it remains unclear which equipment is the most effective. Nebulized pentamidine may cause bronchospasm and patients are therefore pre-treated with a bronchodilator. This is usually nebulized but it may be sufficient in some cases to give the bronchodilator via an inhaler device. (Using a large-volume spacer device may further increase efficacy.) This is quicker, but should always be monitored and only given to those people not developing a significant reduction in peak flow or FEV_1 (Forced Expiratory Volume in one second).

The nebulization of pentamidine should ideally be carried out in a well-ventilated room for reasons of hygiene and possibility of contamination [7]. Patients who administer their own pentamidine at home are fully warned and supervised before being allowed to so do.

Positions for pentamidine delivery

It has been suggested that because of the recurrence of PCP in the apices that the person receiving the pentamidine should lie in a semi-recumbent position, with the legs flexed and fully supported [6]. Alternatively it has been suggested that treatment should be alternated between supine (lying on the back) and upright sitting. A study to investigate effect of body position on pentamadine distribution found that there was a more uniform distribution of pentamidine when it was inhaled in the supine position with a slow and deep inspiration from functional residual capacity, i.e. patients should breath out fully and take a deep breath in from maximum expiration [8]. Compromises may have to be made in the position of the patient if coughing becomes a problem or if the nebulizer equipment does not work effectively on its side.

Adverse reactions to pentamidine

Patients sometimes report that pentamidine has an unpleasant taste. In addition it can induce coughing, increase salivation and cause bronchospasm. Patients should be encouraged to turn off the nebulizer while coughing or expectorating excess saliva. Provision of sweets may make the taste more palatable and those patients with significant bronchospasm may need an additional bronchodilator.

Adjuncts to diagnosis

Early diagnosis of PCP is important and thus recognition of signs and symptoms of infection is vital for patients and carers alike. Since routine investigations may be normal in early PCP, the procedures for a definitive diagnosis are usually bronchoscopy with broncho-alveolar lavage. However, induced sputum and exercise desaturation tests (Chapter 2) are also used to help diagnosis as they are relatively non-invasive, quick and inexpensive to perform. These tests are relatively non-invasive, quick, and inexpensive to perform and thus can be employed as a first line of investigation. If positive results are obtained they may help to avoid more invasive techniques like bronchoscopy and broncho-alveolar lavage.

Sputum induction

As patients with PCP often present with dry non-productive coughs, sputum induction can be useful in providing specimens for investigation. It simply describes a process whereby a productive cough is induced in order to examine the sputum under microscope (Table 4.1).

Contra-indications to sputum induction

Sputum induction should not be performed on people who are severely hypoxic or who have pleural effusions due to Kaposi's sarcoma or lymphoma of the lung. Fatal adverse reactions have been reported in patients with pleural effusions who have undergone sputum induction [12]. It therefore seems prudent to check

Table 4.1 Procedure for sputum induction

The sputum induction is ideally performed in the morning prior to eating in order to avoid contamination of the culture with food.

1. The patient is requested to brush their teeth and mouth with water using a clean toothbrush to minimize contamination.
2. The patient breathes in hypertonic saline (3%) via an ultrasonic nebulizer. The amount needed and time taken are variable: 20–40ml saline, 10–40 minutes.
3. The patient breathes normally, taking in occasional deep breaths and they are encouraged to cough at regular intervals. Teaching the patient the Forced Expiration Technique (FET) may also assist expectoration [9].
4. Two specimens should be collected if possible and labelled '1' and '2'. As the second specimen is thought to contain sputum from a deeper origin, this may give a higher yield of cysts.
5. Sputum specimens are sent to the laboratories to be examined for pneumocystis cysts and any other suspected infections. The reported sensitivity of induced sputum for PCP varies greatly from centre to centre [10,11].

the chest X-ray for pleural effusion prior to undertaking this procedure. Inducing sputum may also cause bronchospasm and arterial desaturation in HIV positive individuals and should be used with care on people with known increase in airway reactivity [13].

Exercise desaturation tests

Exercise desaturation tests may be a useful additional diagnostic indicator in those patients presenting with early symptoms of PCP. The patient is requested to cycle for 5–10 minutes on a cycle ergometer and oxygen saturations are recorded using a pulse oximeter. This is most sensitive if the person cycles vigorously for 10 minutes. A drop in oxygen saturation below 90% is significant. It may help to indicate PCP in those patients complaining of shortness of breath but who may have no significant chest X-ray changes and whose resting arterial blood gases are normal. Unfortunately other pneumomias such as CMV (Chapter 2) may produce a similar pattern of 'exercise desaturation' which limits the usefulness of this investigation [14].

Acute phase physiotherapy treatment of PCP

In the acute phase of PCP, patients may be profoundly hypoxic. The main aims of therapy in this condition are to decrease hypoxia and the resulting symptoms of breathlessness in order to support the patient. Patients with PCP rarely present with sputum retention and so physiotherapy techniques aimed at clearance of sputum are rarely indicated. The following physiotherapy techniques may benefit patients with breathlessness.

Positioning

Correct positioning aims to decrease the work of breathing and maximize the ventilation/perfusion match within the lungs, that is, to enhance the efficiency of respiration and increase oxygen uptake. The best positions for the patient include high side lying, high sitting and forward lean sitting. Optimal positions for individual patients can be assessed by using a pulse oximeter and by monitoring the patient for signs of clinical improvement.

Relaxation

Patients understandably may become very anxious – relaxation, explanation and breathing control may help patients to cope with this frightening condition (Chapter 3).

Breathing exercises

Initially, teaching patients a relaxed breathing pattern may be of benefit though severely hypoxic patients will probably gain more from correct positioning than trying to slow down their breathing pattern. Deep breathing exercises may be of use in the less acute period although many patients complain that they are unable to expand their lungs due to pain and stiffness in the lungs themselves. Adequate analgesia is important.

Oxygen therapy

Appropriate methods of oxygen delivery and humidification are important when supplemental oxygen is needed.

Continuous positive airway pressure (CPAP)

In cases of severe hypoxia, continuous positive airway pressure (CPAP) has been found to be helpful in some patients with PCP [15]. The effects of CPAP are to reduce the work of breathing, increase collateral ventilation and increase the functional residual capacity. By increasing functional residual capacity, collapse of the small airways may be avoided thus improving the ventilation in poorly or non-ventilated alveoli [16]. The advantage of using CPAP on patients in this group who develop respiratory failure is that it may avoid intubation and artificial ventilation. CPAP may be used in the intensive care unit or on the ward. Sometimes it is less distressing for the patient to receive CPAP on the ward so long as close monitoring is maintained.

Complications of CPAP

- *Barotrauma*:
  People with PCP are more at risk of pneumothoraces. Any sudden increases in shortness of breath should be investigated.
- *Decreased cardiac output*:
  This may result from increased intra-thoracic pressure. Close monitoring is essential.
- *Hypoventilation and CO_2 retention*.
- *Mask discomfort and pressure areas*:
  Granuflex can be used over bony points to avoid pressure from the mask.
- *Gastric distension and discomfort due to swallowing of air*.
- *Aspiration of gastric contents*:
  The nasal mask is more appropriate if gastric reflux is a problem.
- *Claustrophobia*:
  It is important to give clear explanation of the treatment's rationale to patients, and to help them to tolerate the mask in the early stages. If CPAP is applied sensitively and tolerated

until the oxygen saturation increases people often find it very helpful. A nasal mask is less claustrophobic and allows the patient to communicate with greater ease.

• *Dryness of mouth and airways*:
   In the short term, adequate oral hydration and care may be sufficient; in the long term, humidification of the circuit may be necessary.

Ventilation

Some patients who develop respiratory failure will be ventilated. This is still associated with a high mortality although centres that regularly treat PCP are reporting improved survival of patients following intubation and ventilation [17]. Physiotherapy treatment of ventilated patients will depend on assessment findings. Again positioning to improve ventilation/perfusion ratios and maximize the efficiency of ventilation may be of benefit. Suctioning or manual hyperinflation (bagging) should only be used if assessment indicates a need. The lungs of these patients characteristically lose compliance and therefore require a high level of positive pressure in order to maintain oxygen saturations. An effort to maintain this level and the oxygenation should be made if suctioning or bagging are indicated. Atelectasis (lung collapse), consolidation and pneumothoraces may also complicate the pneumonia. As with other ventilated patients, joint and muscle stiffness can result from long-term immobility. Passive movements are therefore important in the more long-term ventilated.

Recovery/rehabilitative phase

After an episode of PCP there may be some residual shortness of breath, muscle-wasting and cardiovascular de-conditioning. It is therefore useful to commence patients on gently progressive exercise regimes as soon as the acute illness has subsided. These patients have been shown to benefit from progressive resistance exercise programmes [3]. It is beneficial to show patients who are short of breath on exertion, relaxed and controlled breathing during and after exercise.

Infection control: sputum

Sputum has a very low viral content (although it may contain many other pathogens) and therefore is an inefficient transmitter of the virus. However, if there is blood in the sputum the virus will be present in greater quantities. During endotracheal suction there is a risk of trauma to the bronchial mucosa which may cause blood to mix with the bronchial secretions. The risk to health care personnel stems from the possibility of aerosolised droplets either being inhaled or contaminating other mucosal surfaces [18]. Protective eye wear, masks and latex gloves should therefore be mandatory when suctioning patients. Standing behind a patient while they are coughing is a sensible precaution.

NEUROLOGICAL DISORDERS

In early and late HIV infection neurological problems affecting the nervous system are common. Patients may present to physiotherapy with a variety of neurological syndromes including hemiplegia, peripheral neuropathy, spastic paraplegia, flaccid paraplegia, quadriplegia, ataxia, weakness, sensory disturbance and loss of vision as well as various painful syndromes.

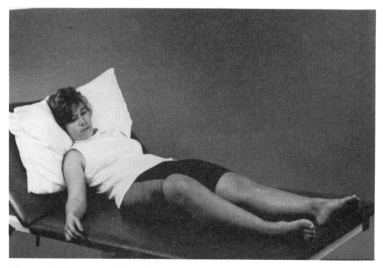

Figure 4.5 Poor position for neurological patients, to be avoided if possible.

Physiotherapy treatment will aim to minimize any discomfort patients may be experiencing and maximize their functional ability where possible (Fig. 4.5). Helping patients to adjust to limitations in physical ability is also another aim where total recovery is not possible.

Although the aims of treatment are the same as for other neurological conditions, the potential progressive nature of AIDS-related complications makes this particularly challenging. Communication with the patient and flexibility in approach is of great importance in order to help the patient achieve his set goals. Lengthy physiotherapy sessions may not always be the most productive use of the patient's time and limited energy resources. The physiotherapy treatment given will depend on the assessment findings and will need to be modified in the light of the patient's condition. Treatment philosophies in physiotherapy differ according to whether the symptoms are those of upper or lower motor nerve pathology. In upper motor nerve lesions as in hemiplegia or in spinal cord lesions, the main problems tend to be those of abnormal co-ordination of movement and posture [19]. Postural tone is altered and often increased, causing resistance to normal movement (spasticity). This movement loss is not due specifically to muscle weakness and so strengthening exercises are not indicated. This should be explained to the patient who may be frustrated to be told to stop strengthening exercises without adequate explanation. The type of physiotherapy approach most commonly used in the UK for upper motor neurological problems is called the Bobath approach [19]. Other approaches to treatment include the motor re-learning programme, conductive education and the Johnstone concept of rehabilitation [20–22].

In lower motor nerve lesions there is specific muscle weakness. Strengthening exercises, facilitation, stimulation and support are indicated in an effort to improve muscle power and function. In HIV infection combinations of upper and lower motor nerve lesions may coexist. Regular and thorough assessment will indicate what kind of treatment will benefit the patient. Rapid fluctuations in the patient's neurological status may occur, necessitating complete reappraisal of aims and goals of treatment. This can be frustrating for the patient as well as the therapist.

Central nervous system

Hemiplegia

Hemiplegia in HIV infection may result from toxoplasmosis, lymphoma, Progressive Multifocal Leucoencephelopathy (PML), infarctions and other infections. Symptoms of hemiplegia may include unilateral impairment of sensation and co-ordination and lateration in the muscle tone on one side of the body. These symptoms may be so mild that they are only obvious when very fine movements are undertaken or they may be so severe that the patient is unable to sit unaided (Fig. 4.6).

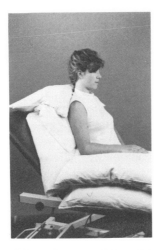

Figure 4.6 Correct position: sitting upright with arm supported in a patient with hemiplegia.

In toxoplasmosis, recovery is usually good and neurological problems often improve following medical treatment (Chapter 2). Physiotherapy may therefore be used to guide the patient through recovering symptoms. However sometimes hemiplegia, ataxia or other neurological signs may result as a lasting deficit. In these cases physiotherapy (with occupational therapy) is important, assisting the patient in gaining maximum functional independence. Occasionally these patients develop severe spasticity necessitating considerable physiotherapy intervention (Fig. 4.7).

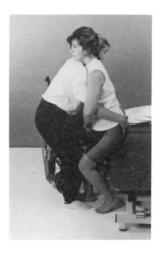

Figure 4.7 Transferring a patient with hemiplegia.

PML is a sub-acute or chronic progressive illness which may present with hemiparesis, ataxia or dementia (Chapter 2). Unlike toxoplasmosis, it does not respond well to treatment and has a poor prognosis. Physiotherapy therefore should work primarily towards maintaining function and symptom control.

Ataxia

Ataxia may result from a wide range of neurological pathologies in HIV infection. Ataxia simply means unsteadiness and incoordination and has many causes. Ataxia resulting from cerebellar disease presents with low muscle tone, inco-ordination and intention tremor. Lack of co-ordination which has a sensory origin (that is, sensory ataxia) may also occur in HIV in peripheral neuropathy and spinal cord pathology. Ataxia is very distressing for patients who find they are unable to co-ordinate movements, especially fine ones. Balance is poor and patients feel unstable and vulnerable when walking. This can be exacerbated further by any deterioration in vision. In cerebellar lesions there is a lack of postural stability [20]. Physiotherapy treatment will need to work at improving proximal stability and balance reactions in order to facilitate normal movement. The provision of a walking aid such as a rollator frame may enhance confidence and improve overall mobility.

Spinal cord disorders

Spinal cord disorders in patients with AIDS is not uncommon [23]. Vacuolar myelopathy is the most common cause of spinal symptoms in HIV infection with symptoms of progressive spastic paraplegia (Chapter 2). Vacuolar myelopathy often coexists with AIDS dementia complex. Patients may require physiotherapy for a variety of symptoms including: mild or severe weakness in the legs, ataxia, back pain, sensory problems, flaccid paraplegia, progressive spastic paraplegia and quadriplegia. These symptoms may be slow or acute in their onset. Peripheral neuropathies may also present with symptoms of paraplegia, although these will demonstrate lower motor neurone signs.

Acute neurological signs – early physiotherapy treatment

Different physiotherapy regimes will be dependent on the type of patient, the cause of the patient's impairment and the aims of the treatment. There are however a number of basic principles of such therapy (Table 4.2).

Table 4.2 Aims of physiotherapy

- Inhibition of abnormal reflex spastic patterns, i.e. normalize muscle tone
- Prevention of contractures
- Prevention of pressure areas developing
- Facilitation of normal movement and normal sensory input
- Maximize comfort
- Maximize function
- Facilitate independence
- Establish realistic goals with each individual

Positioning

To prevent damage to unprotected joints, for example the shoulder joint which, in hemiplegia, may lack the normal muscle protection and sensation. Patients are often turned and left lying on the point of their shoulder. If they are unable to alter their position independently they may spend hours lying in this uncomfortable position. By simply teaching carers how to bring the shoulder through into a more comfortable position this can be avoided.

In paraplegia the position of the feet and hips are of particular importance. Contractures in the achilles tendon will develop if good positioning is not maintained. Provision of a bed cradle will minimize the weight of the sheets on the feet which may have been exacerbating problems. In a patient with a flaccid (low muscle tone) paraplegia, a board to hold the feet up in dosiflexion is useful. However, where there is increased muscle tone, this should be avoided as it stimulates the sole of the foot and increases the muscle tone further.

Good positioning also aims to inhibit onset of abnormal postural tone (spasticity) and increase normal sensory input. The position of the patient has a profound effect on the muscle tone. For example, lying on the back can produce an increase in extensor tone and encourages the shoulder and hip to become retracted. This is not desirable – should the patient need to lie on his back careful positioning with pillows under the hemiplegic shoulder and hip will help to avoid these patterns. Lying slouched (half-lying) in the bed is a damaging position though, sadly, a common one.

If patients need to sit in bed then sitting upright in the bed is preferable although sitting out in a chair is better still. Well-supported side lying is a good position for these patients. Positions such as well-supported alternate side lying are not only valuable for early rehabilitation but are also positions of choice for pressure care and chest care. Early sitting and standing are important positions to prevent some of the complications which are associated with prolonged bedrest.

A suitable wheelchair should be provided at the first opportunity in order that the patient can become mobile. Sensitivity in delivery of the wheelchair is needed as it can be very traumatic for the patient who may perceive the wheelchair as evidence of a permanent inability to walk.

Lifting and handling

Early teaching of lifting and handling techniques to all those involved in care is important, especially where volunteers and untrained persons may be helping with lifting and transfers. Appropriate lifting techniques should avoid trauma to unprotected joints. In addition, these techniques are designed to prevent back injuries to the carer and also help to restore some confidence in the patient. This is particularly important if the patient is cared for at home. Transfers that are performed correctly are an important part of rehabilitation, allowing the patient to experience weight bearing while performing activities of daily living. Co-ordination between physiotherapists, occupational therapists, nurses and other carers from any early stage ensures reinforcement of desired movement patterns and avoids poor lifting techniques.

Normal movement and normal sensory input

Physiotherapists aim to help patients re-establish normal movements by encouraging and maximizing function and preventing stiffness and contractures. Where the patient is unable to move his limbs or trunk independently, the physiotherapist may assist with these movements. Passive/assisted movements of the patient's trunk and limbs are important in order to maintain length of soft tissues and mobility of joints, and to avoid stagnation of the circulation. Movement of limbs can also be very comfortable as it increases normal sensory input. Back pain which may accompany spinal symptoms may be exacerbated by hip flexion. The physiotherapist encourages integration of the whole body to gain symmetrical movement rather than encouraging compensation by increased use of unaffected limbs or joints.

More active rehabilitative phase

As soon as the patient is capable, a more active treatment can commence. Bed mobility, transfers, sitting, standing, walking and activities of daily living should be assessed and treatment given as necessary. A joint assessment with an occupational therapist is often valuable.

Standing frames and tilt tables may be useful for patients who are fatigued in order to achieve standing with less energy expenditure. If increased tone is a problem, then position, specific movements and gentle stretching performed by the physiotherapist may help to reduce the spasticity and maintain the length of soft tissues.

If the spine is irritable, then trunk mobility should be avoided and more static upright positions should be adopted. Occasionally, plastering the limbs to achieve optimal positioning may be helpful. Skin integrity however should be carefully monitored if splints or plasters are used.

Wheelchair mobility and transfers should be taught to patients unable to mobilize independently (Chapter 3). In some cases wheelchair independence may be the most appropriate goal of treatment. Pressure care is particularly important for these patients as they may have atrophic skin changes, impaired sensation, weight loss resulting in prominence of bony points, and weakness in the arms making independent pressure relief in the chair difficult. Coexisting dementia will further increase the risk of pressure areas developing. A suitable cushion should therefore be provided and pressure areas should be closely monitored. Bladder and bowel dysfunction can be very distressing for patients and assessment of incontinence is important.

Gait training should commence as soon as sitting and standing balance are sufficient. Long delays in commencing walking in order to achieve a perfect gait may be less appropriate than aiming for function at an earlier phase in treatment. Provision of a walking aid may be of benefit.

With progressive symptoms, deterioration may be inevitable and physiotherapy will aim to maximize function and minimize discomfort. Assisting patients in coming to terms with the loss of functional ability will be of great importance. The patient and their carers should be actively involved in decisions about treatment at all times. A home visit in conjunction with an occupational therapist may be of value, and out-patient or domiciliary physiotherapy should be organized if continued treatment is needed after discharge from hospital (Chapter 3).

Mild or slow onset of symptoms

For many patients symptoms will be chronic and slow in onset, for example, with progressive spastic paraplegia. Admission to hospital may be unnecessary and out-patient physiotherapy will be indicated. Physiotherapy treatment will be aimed at rehabilitation or maintenance of function by:

- regular monitoring of symptoms
- regular stretching by physiotherapist or by friend/family to prevent contractures
- gait re-education
- a specific home exercise programme
- general advice to the person and carers on aspects of daily living and optimizing function.

Walking aids – sticks, crutches, rollator frames, parallel bars – may be useful in facilitating mobility; splints, plasters and other orthoses are also sometimes indicated.

Lower motor nerve dysfunction – peripheral nerve disorders

Peripheral neuropathies are very common at all stages of HIV infection although they may go unnoticed or overshadowed by other problems in patients who are very weak [24]. Progressive peripheral neurological dysfunction has even been reported in 'asymptomatic' HIV positive individuals [25]. The most common peripheral neuropathies are sensory, often resulting in painful or burning paresthesias, particularly in the feet (Chapter 2) [26].

Transcutaneous electrical nerve stimulation (TNS) has been found useful in some cases [27]. TNS has been used either over the area of pain or on specific acupuncture sites. If the feet are hypersensitive an increase in sensory stimulati. in the form of massage, vibration, ice, heat, etc., may help to desensitize the area. Alternatively, decreasing sensory input by fitting cushioned insoles may help to reduce pain whilst walking. Some of the painful neuropathies are very resistant to treatment and are thus a major cause of morbidity for the patient.

Although the symmetrical distal neuropathies are mainly sensory, there may sometimes be a motor component which tends to be distal, resulting in weakness in the intrinsic muscles of the hands or feet. Walking can become disturbed by a combination of sensory and proprioceptive loss, weakness and discomfort. A foot drop splint may improve gait if dorsiflexion is weak or lost, though careful skin care is important to prevent pressure to areas of sensory impairment. Muscular stimulation, facilitation and strengthening are indicated where weakness is evident.

MUSCULO-SKELETAL AND RHEUMATOLOGICAL DISORDERS

Primary disease of the joints and soft tissue is also now recognized in HIV infection and AIDS although the cause is poorly understood. Rheumatic manifestations of HIV and AIDS include: arthropathies, psoriasis, Reiter's syndrome, spondylitis, plantar fasciitis, myalgia and myositis [28, 29]. Arthritis has been reported particularly in the knees and ankles, but also in the shoulders, fingers and spine. Patients with haemophilia may have additional joint problems caused by bleeds into the joints.

Symptomatic treatment of pain in musculo-skeletal problems may be helpful through the use of ice, heat, electrotherapy, manual techniques, mobilization, exercises and hydrotherapy. For patients with poly-arthropathies more general treatment, rest and exercise programmes are needed. Hydrotherapy may be appropriate and valuable in such cases though fatigue levels should be monitored when using the pool. Spinal stiffness and pain are a common complaint through HIV infection. Back pain is particularly common in patients who have systemic illness, perhaps because of the adoption of poor posture. Patients with spinal stiffness may benefit from general back mobility exercises and postural education.

As with many aspects of HIV, assessment of the presenting symptom is often complicated by other coexisting symptoms and it is sometimes difficult to differentiate between signs. For example, when assessing dermatomes or myotomes in spinal assessment, confusion may occur because of coexisting peripheral neuropathy, muscle weakness and wasting unrelated to the spinal symptoms.

Psoriasis, which is sometimes treated by physiotherapists using ultraviolet light is also more common in HIV positive individuals. Interestingly, it has been suggested, in view of the possible immunosuppressive effect of ultraviolet light, that this treatment is not used for patients who are HIV positive [28].

HIV myopathies

Muscle changes in HIV infection are also extremely common although often sub-clinical or overshadowed by neurological or systemic illness. A muscle analysis study of people with AIDS and ARC (AIDS-Related Complex) found that 96% of biopsies showed substantial abnormalities [30]. These included disuse atrophy, infection, inflammation and necrotizing myopathy [31]. These findings are significant especially for the physiotherapist where function and mobility are highly dependent on muscle status of the patient. Clearly there will be limitations in the potential of exercise therapy where there is denervation, necrosis or inflammation. A gentle exercise programme with adequate warm-up is indicated initially as atrophy, inflammation and necrosis could lead to a greater vulnerability in the tissues. The drug AZT (Zidovudine) has also been implicated as a cause of myalgia and myopathy – this may improve spontaneously if the drug is discontinued (Chapter 2) [32].

HIV wasting syndrome

There is often confusion about the definition and diagnosis of the HIV wasting syndrome. The HIV wasting syndrome is defined as involuntary weight loss of greater than 10% of baseline body weight plus either chronic diarrhoea or chronic weakness. Intermittent or constant fever for more than thirty days is also a component of the diagnosis. Patients diagnosed with HIV wasting syndrome have been found to present with insidiously progressive, proximal muscle weakness. Myalgias (muscle pains), particularly in the thighs, are common complaints [33] (Fig. 4.8).

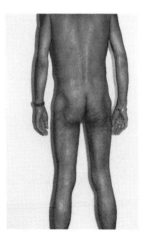

Figure 4.8 Marked muscle wasting in a patient with AIDS.

The effect of exercise on these muscle disorders remains unclear and warrants further investigation. Exercise programmes have however been shown to be effective in patients with muscle atrophy following acute episodes of illness.

Pain accompanying myopathy will inhibit muscle function and limit the success of any exercise programme. Pain should therefore be treated in conjunction with exercise.

Kaposi's sarcoma (KS)

The lesions in Kaposi's sarcoma can be problematic in a number of ways that might involve the physiotherapist. The lesions may be painful, particularly on the soles of the feet where they may affect walking (Fig. 4.9). Symptomatic relief can be gained by the fitting of soft insoles in the shoe or by the provision of a walking aid. If lesions develop around joints, especially where oedema is present, contractures may develop very quickly unless regular stretching exercises are instigated.

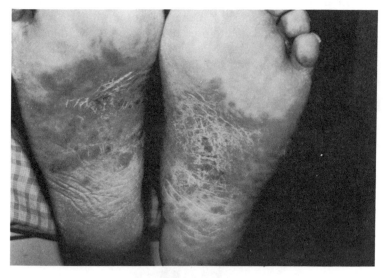

Figure 4.9 Kaposi's sarcoma (KS) involving the feet.

Kaposi's sarcoma commonly involves the lymph nodes where it impedes lymphatic drainage causing oedema. This lymphoedema is seen mainly in the face, lower limbs, abdomen and scrotum (Figs 4.10, 4.11). In the lower limbs, oedema can restrict joint movement and make general mobility difficult. In severe cases the skin may ulcerate. Management of oedema is unsatisfactory yet a major problem for patients with chronic cutaneous Kaposi's sarcoma. Radiotherapy has been useful in treating oedema but can also cause loss of skin elasticity and also loss of movement. All patients need to be monitored closely to maintain range of movement in all joints, ensure skin care and avoid stasis of the circulation. This will help to maintain mobility and independence of the patient.

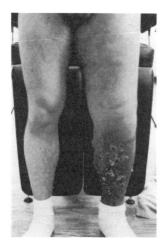 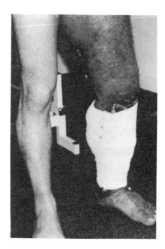

Figures 4.10 and 4.11 Kaposi's sarcoma (KS) showing oedema and flexion contraction at knee.

Controlling lymphoedema

Lymphoedema can be controlled by a number of methods:

- Supply correctly fitted support stockings.
- Avoid prolonged periods of static dependence of the limbs.
- Elevate the limbs when immobile, avoiding excessive flexion at the hip joint.
- Exercises in elevation encourage lymphatic drainage and prevent circulatory stasis.

- Employ manual lymph drainage techniques (a specialized light form of massage aimed at facilitating lymph drainage) [34].
- Use sequential pressure pumps. There is no information to indicate if sequential pressure pumps such as the lymphapress are useful or detrimental to these patients. I found it useful in an individual case where it reduced oedema and improved comfort of the limbs when severe Kaposi's sarcoma and ulceration prevented other manual techniques.

Some of the lymphatic drainage techniques are very time-consuming and patients may prefer to manage lymphoedema at home with support garments and exercises. The value of pressure pumps has yet to be assessed; they may be useful in giving some relief to patients with oedema which is limited to the limbs.

In addition to the control of oedema, the prevention of contractures by regular stretching is very important. Where there is swelling behind the knee, flexion contractures can develop quickly.

Visual impairment

Loss or impairment of vision resulting from cytomegalovirus infection or other neurological infection may lead to diminished confidence and loss of independence and mobility. Assistance with mobility and activities of daily living in conjunction with an occupational therapist is of value in order to maximize the safety and functional independence of a person in their own environment (Chapter 3). Assistance with walking outside with a therapist, carer or volunteer can prevent a person becoming housebound because of loss of vision.

CONCLUSION

Physiotherapy has an important role to play in helping people with HIV infection to maintain, improve and adapt to changes in function and independence. Physiotherapy has traditionally focused on respiratory disorders including the management of pneumocystis carinii pneumonia as well as the acutely ill patient with HIV infection. As the concept of chronicity develops for those with HIV infection, physiotherapists will inevitably become more involved in rehabilitation, prevention of disability and management of pain. Although there is a growing need to assess the value of physiotherapy techniques on a wide variety of HIV-related syndromes, physiotherapy has established itself as a valued member of the multidisciplinary team designed to meet the needs of patients with HIV infection and AIDS.

SUGGESTED READING

Berta, B. *Adult hemiplegia. Evaluation and treatment*, Heinemann medical books, Oxford, 1990.
Bromley, I. *Tetraplegia and Paraplegia. A guide for Physiotherapists.* Churchill Livingstone, London, 1991.
Carr, J.H. and Sheppard, R.B. *Physiotherapy in disorders of the brain. A Clinical Guide*, William Heinmann Medical Books Ltd, London, 1980.
Galantino, M.L. *Clinical Assessment and treatment of HIV. Rehabilitation of a chronic illness*, Slack, New York, 1992.
Hough, A. *Physiotherapy in Respiratory Care. A problem solving approach*, Chapman and Hall, London, 1991.
Johnson, A.J. *Productive living strategies for people living with AIDS*, The Haworth Press, New York and London, 1990.
Lynch, A. and Grisogono, V. *Strokes and Head injuries. A guide for Patients, families and carers*, John Murray (publishers) Ltd, London, 1991.
Mitchell, D. and Woodcock, A. Aids in the Lung. BMJ articles reprinted from *Thorax*, British Medical Journal Publications, London, 1990.
Webber, B.A. *The Brompton Hospital Guide to Chest Physiotherapy*, Blackwell Scientific Publications, Oxford, 1988.

REFERENCES

1. LaPerriere, A.R., *et al.* (1990) Exercise intervention attenuates emotional distress and natural killer decrements following notification of positive serologic status for HIV–1. Biofeedback Self Regulation, **3**, 229–242.
2. Schlenzig, C., *et al.* (1989) Supervised physical exercise leads to psychological and immunological improvement in pre-AIDS patients. Vth International AIDS Conference, (abstract No. TBP 301).
3. Spence, D.W., *et al.* The effect of progressive resistance exercise on muscle function and anthropometry of a select AIDS population. *Archives of Physical Medicine and Rehabilitation*, **71**, 644.
4. Johnson, J., *et al.* (1990) Exercise dysfunction in patients seropositive for the human immunodeficiency virus. *American Review of Respiratory Diseases*, **141**, 618–622.
5. Galantino, M.L. and Spence, D.W. (1988) 'Physical management of HIV patients' in *Nursing Care of the Person with HIV/ARC*. Aspen Publications, Rockville, MD, 186–187.
6. Irvine, M.K. (1991) Nebulised pentamidine for prophylaxis of pneum-

ocystis carinii pneumonia. *The Pharmaceutical Journal*, March 9, HS 24–28.

7. Montgomery, B.A., *et al.* (1990) Occupational exposure to aerosolized Pentamidine. *Chest*, **98**, 2, 386–388.

8. Baskin, M., Abd, A., and Ilowite, J. (1990) Regional deposition of aerosolised pentamadine: Effects of body position and breathing pattern. *Annals of internal medicine*, **113**, 9, 677–683.

9. Partridge, C., Pryor, J., and Webber, B. (1989) Characteristics of the Forced Expiration Technique. *Physiotherapy*, March, **75**, 3, 193–194.

10. Leigh, T., *et al.* (1989) Sputum induction for diagnosis of pneumocystis carinii pneumonia. *Lancet*, **2**, 205–206.

11. Wakefield, A., Guiver, L. and Miller, R. (1991) DNA amplification on induced sputum samples for diagnosis for pneumocystis carinii pneumonia. *Lancet*, **337**, 8754, 1378–1379.

12. Nelson, M.R., *et al.* (1989) Fatal adverse reaction with induced sputum. *Vth International Conference on AIDS*, Abstract 5, 256 (abstract No. MBP 209).

13. Miller, R.F., Bucland, J.G., and Semple, J.G. Arterial desaturation in HIV positive patients undergoing induced sputum. *Thorax*, **46**, 449–451.

14. Smith, D., et al. (1988) Severe exercise hypoxaemia with normal or near normal X-rays: A feature of Pneumocystis carinii infection. *Lancet*, **ii**, 8619, 1049–1051.

15. Kesten, S. and Rebuck, A. (1988) Nasal continuous positive airway pressure in pneumocystis carinii pneumonia. *Lancet*, **i**, 8625, 1414–1415.

16. Miller, R. and Semple, S. (1991) Continuous positive airway pressure ventilation for respiratory failure associated with pneumocystis carinii pneumonia. *Respiratory Medicine*, **85**, 133–138.

17. Efferen, L.S., Nadarajah, D. and Palat, D.S. (1989) Survival following mechanical ventilation fo Pneumocystis carinii pneumonia in patients with acquired immunodeficiency syndrome; a different perspective. *American Journal of Medicine*, **87**, 4, 401–404.

18. Miller, R. and Roberts, C.M. (1991) Intensive Care Management of HIV positive patients and patients with AIDS. *Clinical intensive care*, **2**, 1.

19. Bobath, B. *Adult hemiplegia, Evaluation and treatment*, Heinemann Medical Books Ltd, London, 1990.

20. Carr, J.H. and Shepperd, R.G. *Physiotherapy in disorders of the brain. A Clinical Guide*, William Heinemann Medical Books Ltd, London, 1980.

21. Cottam, P.J. and Sutton, A. *Conductive Education. A system for overcoming motor disorder*, Croom Helm, London, 1986.

22. Johnstone, M. *Restoration of motor function in the stroke patient. A Physiotherapist's approach*, Churchill Livingstone, Edinburgh, 1987.

23. Gray, F., *et al.* (1990) Spinal cord lesions in the Aquired immune deficiency syndrome. *Neurosurgical Review*, **13**, 3, 189–194 (review).

24. Connolly, S. and Manji, H. (June 1991) AIDS and the peripheral

nervous system. Clinical manifestations of AIDS Hospital Update, 474–485.

25. Jakobseen, J., *et al*. (1989) Progressive neurological dysfunction during latent HIV infection. *British Medical Journal*, **299**, 6693, 225–228.
26. Simpson, D.M., Wolfe, D.E. (1991) Neuromuscular complications of HIV infection and its treatment. *AIDS*, **5**, 917–926.
27. Galantion, M.L. and Levy, K.J. (1988) HIV Infection: Neurological Implications for rehabilitation. *Clinical management in physical therapy*, **8**, 1.
28. Foster, S.M., Seifert, M.H., and Keat, A.C. (1988) Inflammatory joint disease and human immunodeficiency virus infection. *British Medical Journal*, **296**, 6637, 1625–1627.
29. Rowe, I.F., *et al*. (1989) Rheumatological lesions in individuals with human immunodeficiency virus infection. *Quarterly Journal of Medicine*, **73**, 272, 1167–1184.
30. Gabbai, A.A., Schmidt, B., and Castello, A. (1990) Muscle biopsy in AIDS and ARC: analysis of 50 patients. *Muscles and Nerves*, **13**, 6, 541–544.
31. Monika, A., *et al*. (1990) Skeletal Muscle Pathology in AIDS: An autopsy study. *Muscles and Nerves*, 13:508–515.
32. Marinos, C., *et al*. (1990) Mitochondrial Myopathy caused by long-term Zidovudine therapy. *New England Journal of Medicine*. April 19, **322**, 1098–1105.
33. Simpson, D.M., *et al*. (1990) Human Immunodeficiency virus wasting syndrome may present a treatable myopathy. *Neurology*, **40**, 535–538.
34. Einfeld, H. (1989) Lymph drainage therapy in secondary lymphoedema caused by Kaposi's sarcoma. *Lymphology*, **13**, 1, 19–22 (review).

5

Nutrition in HIV disease

Carolyn Summerbell

NUTRITIONAL SUPPORT IN ASYMPTOMATIC HIV DISEASE

The rationale for giving advice on diet in asymptomatic HIV disease is based on avoiding nutritional deficiencies and toxicities which may have an impact on immune function, maintaining body weight, and avoiding food and water poisoning. Indeed, the two questions dietitians are most likely to be asked are 'Is there an anti-HIV diet?' and 'What weight should I be?' in terms of keeping well. Unfortunately, we don't know the answer to either of these questions, although we can make certain suggestions from data based around other areas of work.

Dietary components

Most individuals assume that they should be conforming with the 'healthy eating' messages directed at the general population [1]. However, there is little evidence that a low-fat/high-fibre type of diet can improve immune function and thus benefit people with HIV infection. Furthermore, since 'healthy eating' guidelines are, in part, aimed at reducing overweight in the general population, they may indeed be detrimental to the group of individuals affected by HIV disease. The most important aspects of diet for these individuals are that it should not promote weight loss and that it should be enjoyable. In terms of altering immune function, certain aspects of diet may be important and are discussed below.

In general terms, deficiencies and excesses of specific nutrients are known to affect the function of various components of the immune system and influence the resistance to infection [2]. In terms of specific nutrients, vitamins and minerals have attracted the greatest amount of interest.

Vitamins and minerals

There is some evidence that doses of the antioxidant nutrients (Vitamin A, Beta-carotene, Vitamin C, Vitamin E and Selenium) above those recommended for the general population can enhance certain components of the immune system. The basis for this argument comes from the knowledge that in infection, inflammation, stress and trauma, free radical production is increased and thus the requirements for these antioxidant nutrients are raised. However, the efficacy and outcomes of such interventions have not been established using controlled clinical trials.

Regardless, megadoses of these nutrients have been advocated for HIV positive patients to restore cell-mediated immunity by increasing T-cell numbers and activity. Indeed, the amount and availability of information on the use of various vitamins and minerals for HIV positive patients is unprecedented compared to any other client-group. These claims seem to be effective since many of those affected appear to consume large quantities of these nutrients [3,4]. However, when one looks for the justification behind these claims in terms of altered nutritional status as a result of HIV disease, one finds poorly controlled studies and controversy.

Body stores and circulating levels of several vitamins and minerals are recognized as indicators of nutritional status. Several investigators have assessed the vitamin status of subjects at various stages of HIV infection. Folate, Vitamin B6 and Vitamin B12 are the three vitamins that have been studied most frequently and deviations from normal values have been found. However, deviations from normal values have been reported in both directions for each vitamin. These conflicting results are inevitably attributable to several factors, including methods of assessment.

Turning to minerals, a possible association between zinc deficiency and AIDS was suggested relatively early in the history of this epidemic, and generated considerable interest. Subsequent studies have also shown low levels of plasma selenium and raised levels of plasma copper within this patient group. Although these patients may well have a depleted mineral status due to HIV infection, these observations of altered levels of plasma minerals do not provide proof of a deficient intake. As part of the body's response to infection, a defence mechanism called the **acute phase response** occurs.

This response causes alterations in various plasma proteins; albumin declines and caeroplasmin rises. As a consequence, plasma zinc and selenium, which travel in the blood with albumin, decline, while plasma copper which travels with caeruloplasmin, rises. The body's total stores of minerals are not altered, but simply redistributed.

In summary, faced with having to make recommendations using existing evidence, the dietitian should ensure that the diet of the asymptomatic HIV positive individual is adequate in terms of vitamin and mineral content, and if this is in doubt, then supplementation should be advised. A dietary assessment is also useful in ensuring that the client is not consuming megadoses of vitamins or minerals. There may well be a case for recommending extra supplemention of the antioxidant nutrients in the future, but there is not enough evidence available at the moment.

Lipids and amino acids

Modification of the lipid profile of the diet may enhance the immune system. Existing evidence suggests that linoleic acid in excess is immunosuppressive, whereas the omega–3 fatty acids may improve cell-mediated immune response. Indeed, such evidence has already been taken up by certain manufacturers of enteral feeds.

Regarding amino acids, excess arginine is thought to increase thymus size and the number of T-lymphocytes, suppress tumour growth and decrease the incidence of infection. Such optimism also surrounds the amino acid glutamine, and we can probably expect enteral feeds to be modified along these lines in the future.

Specific diets

Because of the seemingly irreversible and inevitable course of HIV disease and AIDS, the lack of a curative therapy, and the natural desire of many to control their own treatment, patients with HIV infection are particularly susceptible to the claims made by proponents of unproven therapies [5,6]. The usefulness of such therapies might be judged against the potential psychological benefit gained from following a particular treatment.

Patients should not be discouraged from following a regime of their choice but helped to evaluate and adjust their chosen eating habits in order to meet nutritional goals. It is important that eating remains an enjoyable experience. The following examples of such therapies are those which are particularly popular among those with HIV infection. Comprehensive reviews of these therapies are available elsewhere [1,5,6].

AL721 is a compound composed of three active lipids (hence AL) mixed in a ratio of 7:2:1. This compound extracts cholesterol from cellular membranes, thus making it more difficult for the virus to attach to receptor sites by increasing membrane fluidity. Preliminary studies in patients have suggested some beneficial effects, and AL721 was approved by the US Food and Drugs Administration for clinical trials in the US. However, in an open label dose ranging trial of AL721 in 40 patients, no consistent trends in T-cell numbers were observed [7].

A macrobiotic diet is based on Oriental philosophy and is purported to restore balance and harmony between yin and yang forces and thereby ameliorate disease. The diet is very low in fat and high in fibre; 50% by volume whole grain cereals, 20–30% vegetables, 10–15% cooked beans or seaweed and 5% miso (fermented soya paste) or tamari broth soup. 'Dr Berger's Immune Power Diet' and the 'Gerson Therapy' are also popular, and contain an abundance of grains, fruits and vegetables. The Gerson Therapy also advocates regular coffee enemas. The major problem with these three special diets for this patient group is that they are inevitably low in calories and this can promote weight loss. However, it is interesting to note that they all contain large quantities of some of the antioxidant nutrients.

The anti-candida diet excludes high-carbohydrate and yeast-containing foods and is purported to prevent opportunistic yeast infections such as candida. Although many patients report an improvement in their oral and oesophageal thrush when adhering to this diet, a controlled trial has never been conducted. Again, one of the problems of this diet is its potential for being low in calories and thus promoting weight loss.

The use of herbs has been advocated as an alternative treatment strategy for HIV infection. A recent study has highlighted the problems of using various herbs in this client-group [8]. Patient care and clinical trials could be distorted because the pharmacological effects of herbs can resemble commonly occurring symptoms in HIV disease as well as side-effects of prescribed or investigational medications.

Finally, certain foods such as garlic and live yoghurt are extremely popular among certain patients with chronic HIV infection. Garlic has been credited with unique antiviral, antiparasitic characteristics and has been used in Chinese medicine for the treatment of cryptococcal meningitis. In a small uncontrolled study of patients with HIV infection certain components of the immune system improved after consuming 10g daily for 12 weeks.

Food and water safety

As in all immunocompromised individuals, food and water safety is extremely important. Work recently carried out on a series of 313 AIDS patients with diarrhoea attributable to a specific pathogen showed that salmonella was the pathogen responsible in 36 of these patients (12%) and cryptosporidium in 99 patients (32%) (personal communication).

Food-borne infections can be prevented by following simple rules of hygiene. Each individual, regardless of the reason for referral to the dietitian, should be given information on the safe handling and cooking of food as well as general good hygiene practices.

Cryptosporidium occurs naturally in drinking water and its concentration varies seasonally. Incidence of cryptosporidium seen in patients mirrors this seasonal variation. The safest method of drinking water is to boil and cool it. This water can then be stored in bottles in the fridge for later use. However, if this is not acceptable we recommend carbonated bottle water, obtained from underground wells. There is some evidence that carbonation has an antibacterial activity, and an analysis of different waters showed that water obtained from springs contained higher bacterial counts compared to those from underground wells [9].

Other problems

Finally, we very often see asymptomatic individuals experiencing financial, social and psychological problems which are in some way affecting their food intake. Possible reasons range from losing one's job because of social stigma at work, to clinical depression over the prospect of a premature death. Eating disorders such as anorexia nervosa are seen more commonly in this patient group compared to the general population [10]. A truly multidisciplinary approach often means a joint assessment of the person with another member of the team or a referral for expert advice. Like most of the multidisciplinary group involved with people who are HIV positive, a significant proportion of the dietitian's time is involved in counselling and support. Being diagnosed as having a life-threatening disease often leaves people feeling out of control. Following the initial shock people often seek strategies for maintaining and promoting health. Food choice is a facet of management in which a person can exert control. Dietary advice should not threaten that control but seek to optimize food intake and achieve nutritional adequacy within the limits of personal choice and social circumstances.

NUTRITIONAL SUPPORT IN ADVANCED HIV INFECTION

Malnutrition is a predominant feature of symptomatic HIV disease, particularly in AIDS-related complex (ARC), and AIDS itself [11]. An average weight loss of 16% from pre-illness weight to death has been observed [12]. Furthermore, malnutrition is a major source of morbidity in patients with infection independent of immune deficiency, [13] and reduces the quality of life experienced by this group. The cause of malnutrition is multifactorial and reflects the variety of symptoms and infections that these individuals may suffer [14]. The correct diagnosis and treatment of any underlying disease is of prime importance in attempting to reverse the malnutrition [15]. In advanced HIV infection, the major causes of weight loss include reduced food intake, altered metabolic requirements and malabsorption. Symptoms associated with HIV disease which can have a potent effect on nutritional status are summarized in Table 5.1.

To date, there is no evidence that reversing the malnourished state alters the course of the disease [2]. However, the deleterious effect of malnutrition on immune function is well-documented in non-AIDS patients and therefore it must be prudent to avoid compromising the immune system further [16]. This nutritional support should be highly individualized to correct for nutritional deficiencies as much as possible in line with patient acceptability, tolerance and socio-economic circumstances (Table 5.2). It is important that other members of the care team are aware of the importance of nutritional support in HIV infected patients. The aims of nutritional support in symptomatic HIV infection are:

- to provide adequate levels of all nutrients
- to achieve/maintain ideal body weight
- to provide symptomatic relief.

On referral, the dietitian will make an initial assessment of nutritional status which should be repeated at regular intervals. The composition of the diet and the most effective route of administration is dependent on the nutritional status, presenting symptoms and stage of disease of the patient. Since patients often have periods of relative well-being between infections, this remission time should be used to optimize nutritional repletion (Chapter 2).

Diarrhoea and malabsorption

These symptoms are caused by gastrointestinal micro-organisms, antibiotic therapy, AIDS enteropathy or malnutrition itself [18].

Some infections of the gastrointestinal tract such as candida, herpes simplex virus and salmonella can be effectively treated. Other opportunistic infections such as cryptosporidium are more resistant to treatment and this may result in profuse diarrhoea, limiting absorption and causing weight loss. Dietary treatment is aimed at relieving symptoms and improving nutritional status where possible. In all cases, increased fluid intake should be encouraged to maintain hydration [20].

A low-fat, low-lactose diet may be useful if steatorrhoea is present, or a low-fibre diet if there is gastrointestinal inflammation or ulceration [21]. However, in many cases dietary restrictions may be of little benefit. If malabsorption is present the use of an elemental or peptide feed should be considered either as a supplement or as a source of total nutrition [12]. Total Parenteral Nutrition (TPN) may be used if a period of bowel rest would relieve symptoms (see table 5.2 for other common problems and their management).

Disorders of the upper gastrointestinal tract

Oral and oesophageal complications of AIDS are common, and result in chewing and swallowing problems and altered taste perception. Causes include infective or malignant lesions of the mouth or oesophagus (e.g., candidiasis, cytomegalovirus, Kaposi's sarcoma) and sometimes regime's treatment (e.g., radiotherapy) [22]. In one study, 94% of people with AIDS had oral candidiasis causing sore mouth and reduced saliva secretion. Effective treatments are available for most of these problems so dietary modification is necessary only until symptoms subside.

Neurological problems

Central nervous system involvement in AIDS ranges from psychomotor retardation to severe dementia [19]. Encephalopathy may be caused by the HIV virus itself or opportunistic infections such as toxoplasmosis or cytomegalovirus encephalitis (Chapter 2). Symptoms include memory difficulties, apathy, short concentration span and impaired ability with tremor [17]. All these factors further reduce the individual's capacity to maintain an adequate nutritional intake.

Tiredness and depression

Some people may be too tired or unmotivated to shop or cook for themselves. The effect of this on nutritional intake is significant and should not be underestimated.

Night sweats and fevers

Night fevers and sweats are a common feature of HIV disease although their cause is unknown. However, these symptoms have nutritional implications in terms of replacing fluids and salts.

ENTERAL AND PARENTERAL NUTRITION

Enteral feeding and Total Parenteral Nutrition (TPN) have been shown to be effective in reversing weight loss associated with HIV infection, particularly when malabsorption is the main feature in the absence of systemic infection [23–26].

Enteral feeding

Sip feeds

Where patients cannot achieve adequate nourishment using normal foods, intake should be supplemented with or replaced by

Table 5.1 Common manifestations of AIDS and associated nutritional problems

AIDS-related infections and cancers	Associated nutritional problems
Opportunistic infections	
Fungal:	
Candida Oral	Sore mouth, altered taste perception, anorexia, reduced saliva production
Candida Oesophageal	Dysphagia
Cryptococcus Meningitis	Pyrexia, nausea and vomiting
Protozoan:	
Toxoplasmosis	Pyrexia, lethargy, confusion
Pneumocystis carinii pneumonia (PCP)	Pyrexia, dyspnoea, anorexia and weight loss, tiredness and lethargy
Bacterial:	
Mycobacterium avium-intracellulare (MAI)	Pyrexia, anorexia and weight loss, diarrhoea and malabsorption
Viral:	
Cytomegalovirus (CMV)	Pyrexia, diarrhoea and malabsorption
Herpes simplex (Oral)	Sore mouth, dysphagia, ulcers
Human immunodeficiency virus (HIV)	Pyrexia, diarrhoea and weight loss
Parasitic:	
Cryptosporidium	Diarrhoea and malabsorption, anorexia, weight loss, nausea and vomiting, pyrexia
Cancers:	
Kaposi's sarcoma	Dysphagia, sore mouth, anorexia, abdominal discomfort and obstruction, diarrhoea and malabsorption
Non-Hodgkin's lymphoma	Anorexia, weight loss, dysphagia, and diarrhoea
Other:	
AIDS enteropathy	Diarrhoea and malabsorption, weight loss
AIDS encephalitis	Confusion, dementia, lethargy

Table 5.2 Dietary management of common AIDS-associated nutritional problems

Symptom	Management
Anorexia	High-calorie, high-protein diet, nutrient-dense supplements, eat little and often; encourage favourite foods; flexible timing of meals; nutritious snacks and convenience foods; appetite stimulant (e.g. megestol acetate); check other drug interactions and change medication times if indicated; nasogastric or gastrostomy feeding.
Nausea and vomiting	Use anti-emetics or alter timings of anti-emetic medication; small, frequent meals; drink plenty of fluids; avoid drinking with meals; avoid cooking smells; avoid rich, fatty and spicy foods; try plain, dry or salty foods; have food cool or cold rather than hot; encourage nutrient-dense supplements; relax when eating; do not lie down after eating.
Neurological problems	Close monitoring and encouragement of patient; help at mealtimes; involve family, friends, carers; may need home help or meals-on-wheels; involve voluntary organizations if appropriate; in case of motor impairment, provide modified-texture diet and/or consider special utensils.
Tiredness and depression	Involve friends, family, other carers; support through volunteers, home help, meals on wheels, day centres, advice on nutritious convenience and snack foods; encourage supplements.
Diarrhoea and malabsorption	Small, frequent meals, low-fat, low-lactose, low-residue diet; low-lactose nutrient-dense supplements; warm food rather than extremes of hot or cold; elemental or peptide feeding; Total Parenteral Nutrition (TPN) may be indicated.
Sore mouth	Modify texture to suit individual – soft, semi-solid or fluid; moist foods may be easier to manage; avoid spicy, salty, acidic or rough foods; take fluids through a straw; avoid extremes of temperature (cold or warm foods are more soothing and taste better); use nutritionally complete liquids; good oral hygiene is important; may need to consider nasogastric feeding if prolonged.
Dry mouth	Frequent drinks, especially sips of fizzy drinks; avoid too much salt and salty foods, make foods moist with gravy and sauces; try saliva-stimulating pastilles or an artificial saliva spray; keep lips moist with vaseline or lip balm.
Taste changes	Provide a variety of textures, use strong smelling foods, use more herbs and spices; cold foods may taste better than hot; use alternative protein sources, marinading meat may make it taste better; encourage good oral hygiene.

Table 5.2 Dietary management of common AIDS-associated nutritional problems—*continued*

Swallowing problems	Modify texture to individual tolerance – smooth, thick consistency is often best; encourage nutritionally complete supplements; may need to consider nasogastric or gastrostomy feed if dysphagia is very bad.
Night fevers and sweats	Replace fluids and salts.
Blindness	Appropriate management and utensils.

nourishing fluids taken at regular intervals. Commercially manufactured protein and energy supplements are very useful. A range of products and flavours should be offered to avoid taste fatigue.

Tube feeding

If a patient fails to achieve adequate intake orally, nasogastric feeding should be initiated. This may be difficult if the patient has nausea and vomiting or has a severe candida overgrowth of the oesophagus. In gastrointestinal malabsorption states, e.g. cytomegalovirus (CMV), pancreatitis or colitis, elemental feeds which are generally low in fats may be best tolerated. Alternatively, digestive enzyme-replacement capsules may be helpful in such cases.

For long-term feeding, a gastrostomy may be considered [27]. This has the advantage of being more socially acceptable for the individual in terms of self-image, although care must be taken in minimizing infection risk in this immunocompromised patient group.

Ideally, enteral feeds should be:

- low-lactose
- low-residue
- low-fat, if steatorrhoea present
- elemental, if malabsorption severe.

Total Parenteral Nutrition (TPN)

Parenteral nutrition should be reserved for cases when the gastrointestinal tract cannot be used, e.g. total small bowel disease, cryptosporidiosis or CMV inflammation, which gives rise to uncontrolled diarrhoea and malabsorption. In the US, Central Parenteral Nutrition (CPN) and Peripheral Parenteral Nutrition (PPN) are much more frequently used to manage HIV wasting syndrome than in the UK. PPN is used for short-term feeding (7–10 days). For more prolonged feeding a central line is indicated.

It is important to remember that many patients with HIV infection and AIDS obtain their advice and treatment solely from Sexually Transmitted Disease (STD)/HIV clinics and may not have a GP or may choose not to involve their GP. Also, patients may travel a long way to centres for treatment. This raises the question of who prescribes and supplies TPN as well as monitoring and follow-up (Chapters 1 and 7).

IS PALLIATIVE NUTRITIONAL SUPPORT EVER JUSTIFIED?

The role of nutritional support in late HIV disease and AIDS is similar to that in terminal oncology patients. It is sometimes assumed that nutritional support in this group is of little importance and whereas this may be true for some patients, it is not true for all and the potential positive benefits to psychological status should not be forgotten [28].

The difference for people with AIDS is that they may suddenly succumb to a debilitating, life-threatening infection after previously being well or even unaware of their HIV positive status. This rapid onset of end-stage HIV disease may leave a person with little time to tackle personal goals – coming to terms with death; seeing loved ones for the last time; making a will; the wish to die at home. Nutritional support in this context may be used not to increase weight but to stabilize and control symptoms. The result is the extension of effective life so that some of the remaining goals may be realized.

DRUGS USED IN HIV DISEASE

There are many drugs used in the management of HIV infection [29,30]. Drug regimes vary depending on who is prescribing, patient preferences and the results of research trials. Those drugs which may have nutritional consequences are listed in Table 3.

Routine anti-emetics, antidiarrhoeal drugs and appetite stimulants are commonly prescribed in the management of HIV infection. An example of the latter, a synthetic progresterone is

Table 5.3 Potential nutritional consequences associated with drugs used in the management of HIV disease (see Appendix for a more comprehensive list)

AIDS-related infections	Drug treatments	Potential nutritional consequences
Viral:		
HIV	Zidovudine (AZT)	Nausea, vomiting
	Dideoxyinosine[1] (DDI)	Nausea, vomiting, diarrhoea, raised blood glucose, Stevens Johnson's syndrome
Herpes simplex	Acyclovir	Nausea, vomiting, diarrhoea
Cytomegalovirus (CMV)	Ganciclovir	Nausea, vomiting
	Foscarnet	Anaemia, nausea, vomiting, nephrotoxic
	Acyclovir	(as above)
Fungal:		
Candida	Ketoconazole Itraonazole Fluconazole	These three drugs may cause mild nausea, diarrhoea and/or vomiting.
	Nystatin lozenges Amphotericin lozenges	These lozenges cause negligible side effects.
Protozoan:		
Pneumocystis carinii pneumonia (PCP)	Pentamidine	Diarrhoea
	Fansidar (Roche)	Mild nausea after eating
	Dapsone	Mild nausea
	Co-trimoxazole	Nausea, diarrhoea, Stevens Johnson's syndrome
Toxoplasmosis	Fansidar (Roche)	(as above)
Bacterial:		
Mycobacterium avium intacellulare (MAI)	Rifabutin	Nausea, diarrhoea
	Clofazimine	Nausea
Parasitic:		
Cryptosporidium	Azithromycin	Nausea, diarrhoea
	Erythromycin	Nausea
	Spiramycin	Nausea
Cancers:		
Kaposi's sarcoma	Chemotherapy (e.g. Vinblastine) Vincristine	Nausea, vomiting
	Radiotherapy	Depends on site of radiotherapy

megestrol acetate which has been used as an appetite stimulant in the management of weight loss in HIV infection. Initial studies show promising results [31–33]. Beneficial side effects, in terms of weight gain, have been reported with the use of certain antiviral agents, e.g. AZT and Gancyclovir [34–36]. Many patients with HIV infection may be prescribed a combination of the drugs described above. The nutritional consequences of these drug combinations are less clear.

CONCLUSION

Dietetics in relation to the care of individuals with HIV infection and AIDS is a rapidly expanding speciality and forms a significant part of the multidisciplinary team. While the exact nutritional consequences of HIV infection remain undefined, the effects of vitamin and mineral deficiencies and toxicities, depleted body weight, and food and water poisoning may be severe and debilitating. Food intake is an area where individuals can exert direct control on their health and any dietary advice should not undermine this control but work with the client's dietary beliefs and practices.

The aim of dietary advice in symptomatic HIV disease is the management and control of symptoms which result from opportunistic infections associated with the condition. Additionally, many of the medications used in the treatment and management of the disease have side-effects which contribute to symptoms, particularly nausea and reduced appetite. Symptomatic relief by dietary modification can reduce the deleterious effect of reduced food intake, malabsorption and increased metabolic rate on nutritional status. For these reasons the dietitian should be an integral member of the multidisciplinary team in the care and management of patients with HIV infection and AIDS.

REFERENCES

1. Summerbell, C.D., Catalan, J. and Gazzard, B. (1993) A comparison of the nutritional beliefs of Human Immunodeficiency Virus (HIV) seropositive and seronegative gay men. *Journal of Human Nutrition and Dietetics*, **6**, 23–27.
2. Raiten, D.J. (1990) *Nutrition and HIV Infection.* Prepared for the Centre for Food Safety and Applied Nutrition, Food and Drug

Administration, Department of Health and Human Services, Washington, DC 20204, PDA Contract 223–88–2124.

3. Fordyce-Baum, M.K., *et al.* (1990) Toxic levels of dietary supplementation in HIV–1 infected patients. *Archives of Research*, **IV**, 149–157.

4. Hand, R. (1989) Alternative therapies used by patients with AIDS. *New England Journal of Medicine*, **320**, 672–673.

5. Pike, J.T. (1988) Alternative nutritional therapies – Where is the evidence? *AIDS Patient Care*, February, 31–33.

6. Dwyer, J.T., *et al.* (1988) Unproven nutritional therapies for AIDS: What is the evidence? *Nutrition Today*, March/April, 25–33.

7. Mildvan, D., *et al.* (1991) An open-label, dose-ranging trial of AL721 in patients with persistent generalised lymphadenopathy and AIDS-related complex. *Journal of AIDS*, **4**, 10, 945–951.

8. Kassler, W.J., Blanc, P. and Greenblatt, R. (1991) The use of medicinal herbs by Human Immunodeficiency Virus-Infected patients. *Archives of Internal Medicine*, **151**, 2281–2288.

9. Stickler, D.J. (1989) The microbiology of bottled natural mineral waters. *Journal of the Royal Society of Health*, **109**, 118–124.

10. Ramsay, N., Catalan, J. and Gazzard, B. (1992) Eating disorders in men with HIV infection. *British Journal of Psychology*, **160**, 404–407.

11. Chelluri, L. and Jastremski, M.S. (1989) Incidence of malnutrition in patients with acquired immunodeficiency syndrome. *Nutritional Clinical Practice*, **4**, 16–18.

12. Hickey, M.S. and Weaver, K.E. (1988) Nutritional management of patients with ARC or AIDS. *Gastrointestinal Clinics of North America*, **17**, 3, 545–561.

13. Kotler, D.P., *et al.* (1989a) Magnitude of body cell mass depletion and the timing of death from wasting in AIDS. *American Journal of Clinical Nutrition*, **50**, 444–447.

14. Summerbell, C.D., Perrett, J.P. and Gazzard, B.G. (1993) Causes of weight loss in Human Immunodeficiency Virus Infection. *International Journal of STD and AIDS*, **4**, 234–236.

15. Grunfeld, C. and Kotler, D.P. (1991) The wasting syndrome and nutritional support in AIDS. *Seminars in Gastrointestinal Disease*, **2**, 1, 25–36.

16. Chandra, R.K. (1981) Immunocompetence as a functional index of nutritional status. *British Medical Bulletin*, **37**, 1, 89–94.

17. Resler, S. (1988) Nutrition Care of AIDS Patients. *Journal of the American Dietetic Association*, **88**, 828–832.

18. Ghiron, E., Dwyer, L.J. and Stollman, L.B. (1989) Nutrition support of the HIV Positive, ARC and AIDS patient. *Clinical Nutrition*, **8**, 103–113.

19. Winick, M., *et al.* (1989) Task Force on Nutrition Support in AIDS. *Nutrition*, **5**, 1, 39–46.

20. Hyman, C. and Kaufman (1989) Nutritional impact of acquired immune deficiency syndrome: A unique counselling opportunity. *Journal of the American Dietetic Association*, **89**, 520–524.

21. King, A.B., *et al.* (1989) Less diarrhoea in HIV patients on a low fat,

elemental diet. *Vth International Conference on AIDS*, Montreal. Th.B. 300 (Abstract).
22. Barr, C.E. and Torosian, J.P. (1986) Oral manifestations in patients with AIDS or AIDS related complex. *Lancet*, **2**, 288.
23. Janson, D.D. and Feasley, K.M. (1989) Parenteral nutrition in the management of gastrointestinal Kaposi's sarcoma in a patient with AIDS. *Clinical Pharmacology*, **8**, 536–544.
24. Singer, P., *et al.* (1989) Nutrition, the gastrointestinal tract and the acquired immune deficiency syndrome. Facts and Perspectives. *Clinical Nutrition*, **8**, 281–287.
25. Kotler, D.P., *et al.* (1990) Effect of home total parenteral nutrition on body composition in patients with acquired immunodeficiency syndrome. *Journal of Parenteral and Enteral Nutrition*, **14**, 5, 454–458.
26. Kotler, D.P., *et al.* (1991) Enteral alimentation and repletion of body cell mass in malnourished patients with acquired immunodeficiency syndrome. *American Journal of Clinical Nutrition*, **53**, 149–154.
27. Kelson, K., *et al.* (1991) Percutaneous endoscopic gastrostomy feeding in AIDS. *VIIth International Conference on AIDS*, Florence. MB 2414 (abstract).
28. Peck, K., *et al.* (1991) Total parenteral nutrition in palliation of AIDS. *VIIth International Conference on AIDS*, Florence MD 4182 (abstract).
29. Tuazon, C.U. and Labriola, A.M. (1987) Management of infections and immunological complications of AIDS: Current and future prospects. *Drugs*, **33**, 66–84.
30. Erskine, D. (1990) The use of drugs in patients with gastrointestinal manifestations of AIDS. *Bailliere's Clinical Gastroenterology*, **4**, (2), 563–583.
31. Chen, W., *et al.* (1990) A retrospective study on the effect of megace on body weight in HIV infected patients who had lost more than 5% body weight. *VIth International Conference on AIDS*, San Francisco. Th.B. 209 (abstract).
32. Von Roenn, J., *et al.* (1989) Megestrol acetate in the treatment of HIV related cachexia. *Vth International Conference on AIDS*, Montreal. Th.B. 309 (Abstract).
33. Summerbell, C.D., *et al.* (1992). Megestrol acetate vs cyproheptadine in the treatment of weight loss associated with HIV infection. *International Journal of STD & AIDS*, **3**, 278–280.
34. Fischl, M.A., *et al.* (1987) The efficacy of azidothymidine (AZT) in the treatment of patients with AIDS and AIDS related complex. A double blind placebo controlled trial. *New England Journal of Medicine*, **317**, 185–91.
35. Kotler, D.P., *et al.* (1986) Treatment of disseminated cytomegalovirus infection with 9-(1,3 dihydroxy–2-propoxymethyl) guanine: evidence of prolonged survival in patients with AIDS. *AIDS Research*, **2**, (4), 299–307.
36. Kotler, D.P., *et al.* (1989b) Body mass repletion during ganciclovir treatment of cytomegalovirus infections in patients with AIDS. *Archives of Internal Medicine*, 149, 901–905.

6

The social worker's role

Stuart Bairstow

I am a community social worker in London. I work with people with HIV/AIDS. In earlier years I worked in the area of mental health, drug and opiate use, adoption and adolescent fostering. I have also been a full-time trainer and educator in HIV and AIDS awareness.

Sometime ago I had arranged to meet some social work friends in a bar for Sunday lunch. Over the till was a sign about two feet wide with large black writing which said 'Warning: These Premises are protected by a pit bull terrier with AIDS'. At the request of one of my party the sign was removed. I was impressed that the landlord actually listened to our points and appeared to understand why such a sign might be offensive and misleading. This is just one example of the many challenges that HIV and AIDS presents us with. The sign was misleading in its suggestion that HIV could be both present in, and transmissible from, dogs. It was offensive in its suggestion that AIDS equalled fear, aggression and violence.

Many of us who became social workers may have done so because we are 'issues' people and are attracted by challenges like the one I have just described. Indeed, some of us entered social work because we thought it would be a profession that encouraged challenge. Social workers have a reputation for being able to debate issues endlessly. An example of this is the continuing dialogue within the profession about equal opportunities. Throughout the 1980s, social workers turned their attention to equality of opportunity in terms of employment and access to social services. It is perhaps not surprising therefore that the multiplicity of issues connected with HIV and AIDS should have been adopted by some social workers under the general umbrella of equal opportunities.

This growing consciousness has taken place amidst a fundamental shift in thinking about public services. For social work, this has been manifest in the introduction of legislation relating to community care and children. Part of this change is the demand for each of the services to think about its value and even its marketability. The 'value for money' principle has arguably permeated all thinking in the caring professions. We are at risk of evaluating our services in economic terms – how much are we able to provide and how much will it cost? The danger is that we will be distracted from the task of ensuring that services are provided on the basis of need rather than financial dictates.

In Britain the funding arrangements for HIV and AIDS services have been largely based on special grants to health and local authorities. These grants have been given on an annual basis with controls on the ways in which the money could be spent.

Local authorities have had widely differing levels of grant funding. Some have had no funding at all, while the London authorities have had the largest share. The services provided have been of a specialist nature, to some extent determined by this method of finance. This created the notion that people with HIV and AIDS were receiving a 'Rolls Royce' standard of social work and related social services compared to other users such as the elderly. In the early days of the epidemic there were fewer people with AIDS to share what resources there were. In other words, there was more to go around. As the numbers of people with HIV and AIDS using social services increases faster than levels of finance, we have witnessed the contraction of services. In other words, there is not so much to go around. The political climate surrounding HIV/AIDS can become heated, especially during a time when other services to other client-groups are under pressure and in many instances being reduced. Nevertheless, users of HIV/AIDS patient services can sometimes wonder what the money has actually been spent on. It is not always possible to see very clearly what the returns are for each million pounds spent. Many authorities have chosen to deploy significant parts of their grants into creating a variety of different posts in social services including the creation of social work jobs.

It is perhaps not surprising that the work of the HIV social worker will be under scrutiny. Some of the questions that might be asked by those who are responsible for future planning of services are: Does the provision of 'social workers' as a resource to people with HIV and AIDS contribute in any significant way to this service user group? Do social workers in the field have any value, and if so, what is it?

Well, just what is it that social workers do? In simple terms, we care for the social aspects of people's lives, the widely accepted definition of social workers being one of people who care for the poor, the needy and children. The public image of social work will vary and is inconsistent. When child abuse hits the headlines of the tabloid press, social workers are criticized for not having prevented neglect or for acting too hastily in taking children into care. Perhaps social workers are asked to be the conscience of society by taking care of the poor, the homeless and the vulnerable. This is often a contentious issue. The idea that it is a social work task to care for the poor and homeless would, I suspect, be a cause for debate within the profession itself. Nevertheless, many users of social services have little money and poor housing.

The wider discussion about the role of social work and society's expectations of it has relevance to the social worker working with people with HIV/AIDS. Issues which people with HIV/AIDS face are not exclusive to that disease category. For example, some of the people presenting to social services because they have financial and housing difficulties may have HIV/AIDS. Confusion about the role of social workers is not only in the minds of the public but also in the minds of other workers in the caring professions.

Social workers can sometimes give mixed messages to other professionals about whether they will help with problems to do with finance and housing. I will, and do, assist with money and housing matters when I can. Indeed, most of my clients have sought social work help with practical problems relating to these key areas. Very often social workers will help with housing and welfare rights even though they may not think that this should be part of their job.

At the beginning of my work with people with HIV/AIDS, I felt the need to search for the 'tangible'. My previous areas of work had been in adolescent fostering as a worker on a family placement scheme. Although I told myself that any skills I had were transferable to work with people with HIV/AIDS, I was uncertain as to what these skills actually were. I suspected that they would be in areas relating to loss, bereavement and separation. I had run some training courses for foster carers on working with loss and grief, and had participated in HIV courses myself. I was anxious about moving into this new area of work and uncertain about my abilities.

The first piece of work that I was presented with was to assess a man who had been admitted to hospital with a serious debilitating illness related to HIV infection. This had left him unable to walk or use his arms. What, if anything, could a social worker have to offer?

I had been told that he had returned from abroad, had nowhere to live and little money. I consoled myself with the thought that perhaps I could offer some practical assistance. I ran through my mind the welfare benefits he might be able to claim, and thought about possible strategies that I might employ to approach any housing difficulties he may have. Such concrete and tangible things would perhaps increase my purpose and make me feel that I, as a social worker, had some relevance.

This was also to be the first time that I had been on an HIV/AIDS hospital ward. I remember it being very hot. The medical and nursing staff appeared to be very busy and purposeful. I entered a side room to approach Mr Jones, who was looking extremely unwell, had obviously been vomiting, and was connected to tubes. It was clearly not appropriate to ask him if he wanted to apply for a travel permit at this particular time!

How would I initiate a discussion about his needs? I simply told him my name and job and asked if there was any way in which I could help. 'If I manage to get out of here I'll need somewhere to live,' he said. 'I don't have any money either.'

These two presenting problems were to become all too familiar to me as my work with people with AIDS progressed. Also familiar by now was the debate about whether welfare rights work and housing advocacy were appropriate tasks for social workers. So what could I say to him: 'Sorry, I don't deal in welfare rights and housing but I'm good at listening to your feelings'? I took the pragmatic approach and wrote in strict confidence to the principle housing officer of the relevant borough.

I helped him fill out an application form for income support and advised him about other disability benefits that he might claim. By the third interview I had given him information about other services and had put him in contact with a volunteer at the Terrence Higgins Trust. By the eighth week he was discharged from hospital to stay on the sofa-bed at a relative's flat. By the tenth week he was housed in a flat belonging to a housing association.

I had arranged for his social services department to install a telephone. I had approached three charities asking for grants to help him equip his flat which, together with a grant from the Department of Social Security, enabled him to buy a cooker, fridge, washing machine, microwave oven, carpets and a sofa.

His recovery from this, his first opportunistic infection, had been remarkable. It had been better than anyone had expected. His own determination to continue to live life was high. My own sense of achievement was high too. I had not only assisted him in his claim for benefits but raised a considerable amount towards his housing needs. The things that I had done had been measurable and had obvious relevance.

Throughout this period, however, Mr Jones had not talked about mortality, illness, death, dying or mobility. The fact that he had not done so raised questions for me about both my role and skills as a social worker. I could not find a prescription that would tell me what a social worker with people with HIV and AIDS either did, or should do. It seemed like unchartered territory and as such was a matter of opinion. But surely part of my role was to counsel him?

By the third month of my contact with Mr Jones, and still feeling this lack of clarity about my role, Mr Jones made a casual remark to me. 'I don't know about you', he said, 'but don't you find that life before is different to life after?' At first I understood his remark to be a reference to his life before and after AIDS. I thought that he was now ready to talk. As a social worker I would be called upon to use my counselling skills. 'Would you like to say more?' I asked. 'My life has been different since I first had penetrative sex,' he replied! The lesson for me here was to recognise that my agenda of issues relating to illness, death and dying was quite radically different from his which was centred around questions of sex and desirability. Resuming a sexual life was more important to Mr Jones than discussions about his mortality. As a social worker I listened and attempted to facilitate further discussions. This is not to suggest that Mr Jones had difficulty in this area but rather that he had simply chosen to share with me his experiences. It was while working with this man that I became aware that I had made an inaccurate assumption about people with HIV and AIDS, that is, that they necessarily needed therapy and/or counselling.

Mr Jones had been determined to regain his independence. He returned to work abroad. Two years later he returned to Britain with another opportunistic infection. Again he was homeless and had very little money. Two weeks later he died.

If the ability to advocate is a skill, then it is that skill that I brought to bear with Mr Jones. I brought advocacy for the practical issues, advocacy for his housing problem and information about the welfare benefits available. The practical approach was the most pragmatic option for me to pursue.

Had he lived, I would have assisted him again with his housing and benefits. Some health service workers thought him irresponsible to have left the country only to return with the same practical difficulties. Some thought, that as a social worker, I could (and should) have pointed out the 'foolish' choice that he had made in leaving the country after his first illness. I felt I should respect the choice that he had made. It is often tempting to advise people with HIV to make decisions that we think we would make for ourselves. Mr Jones spent the last two years of his life doing what *he* wanted to do. Who are we to make judgments about it?

Developing a non-judgmental attitude towards those we work with confronts us with our own prejudices. Sometimes we may need others to help us see this. A worker was reported as saying to a woman with AIDS that many gay men with HIV who claimed benefits were known to be holidaying in exotic places. Implied in this remark was a degree of disapproval. Did it also suggest that those people with HIV who are not gay *are* deserving of such holidays? Did it imply a hierarchy of people with HIV in terms of those who are deserving and those who are not? Such ideas are often based on notions of guilt and innocence and can be found at the centre of some of the social pressures on some people with HIV and AIDS.

It is necessary for social workers involved in helping people with HIV and AIDS to develop good support systems to understand these social pressures. Social workers should aim not to discriminate on the basis of race, religion, class, culture, gender or sexual preference. They have a significant role to play in supporting people with HIV and AIDS cope with those in their social and support networks, such as family and friends, who *do* discriminate. These aims of countering and challenging discrimination are admirable. However, sometimes such challenges can be experienced as being very persecutory. The atmosphere of 'political correctness' can sometimes feel like an added pressure on new workers to HIV and AIDS. This is not to say that there is anything wrong with confronting prejudice but is not helpful to criticize someone for not 'thinking correctly'.

One way to assist social workers in discovering and dealing with their prejudices is to create educational opportunities. For example, I had been asked to spend a day training home care workers on issues relating to the home care needs of people with HIV/AIDS. In the introductory part of the day, two problems became apparent. First, most of the participants had been sent on the course and would have preferred not to have attended. Second, some of the language that they used would have been considered offensive particularly by people with HIV/AIDS, lesbians and gay men. What were my choices? I could have directly challenged the participants and told them that some of the things they were saying were not acceptable. Furthermore, they were committing disciplinary offences. Alternatively, I could view this situation as an opportunity to explore some of the issues around caring for people with HIV/AIDS. My experience told me that the first course would create a bad atmosphere and reinforce attitudes; choosing a more pragmatic approach could possibly create an opportunity for some self-examination and learning. I found it helpful to share with them some stories about the issues that people with HIV/AIDS had presented. The stories are true. The names of the individuals, places and dates have been changed to preserve anonymity.

> When Ellen was discharged home she needed help each day. After six weeks of living with deteriorating health she telephoned me asking if I could arrange for some respite care on a residential basis. She had been having very disturbed nights because of heavy sweats. At 9.15 a.m., having decided that her request was a priority, I had made two phone calls – one to each of the main centres in London offering respite care. Both of the centres wanted to know quite a lot of detail, some of which was medical. Could a social worker provide this detail, and if they could not, would a referral be accepted? Even if a social worker could provide a medical history, would this be appropriate in any case? Both centres wanted infor-

mation from doctors. I sought assistance from a community liaison nurse based in a team of district nurses at a local health centre. Could she arrange for my client's doctor to send reports? I phoned a doctor at a local treatment centre. She was not available and was not expected until next week. I tried the ward on the hospital; the doctor I needed to speak to was not there either. Later that day, (five hours later), the community nurse located the general practitioner who provided the help we needed.

A 22-year-old man had contacted me to ask if I could assist him in getting a fridge for his room. He told me that he had not been well; because of this I had arranged to visit him at his home. He was living in a one-room flat with an en-suite toilet and bath, and a kitchen that would have been more appropriately described as a cupboard. Nine years ago he had been diagnosed HIV-antibody positive. 'My parents do not contact me now,' he said. 'They are embarrassed about me. My doctors think that I may have a lymphoma on the brain. My thinking is very slow. They said I might have to go into hospital for investigations.'

I visited a man who had lost a great deal of weight. On his legs he had extensive and very visible Kaposi's sarcoma. During proceeding weeks, he had persistent diarrhoea. At the time of my visit he had become constipated and, despite the morphine that was being prescribed for him, was in discomfort. He lived alone. His partner had left him three years before. Before I left he asked me to help him change his bed which had become saturated with sweat from the night before. Each day, a home care assistant visited him for 1½ hours. While on that visit, he told me that he wanted to die at home.

Last week I went to see John, the partner of Alan. Alan is very sick and has been unwell for several months. Alan is now in hospital. John has been finding the situation hard to cope with. He has a full-time job in a private company. His employers do not know that he is gay and neither do his parents. No-one knows that his partner has AIDS. Alan no longer feels like having sex and expresses jealousy over John masturbating.

I recently visited a man who can do very little for himself.

Most of the time he needs help getting dressed and undressed. He has told his elderly mother that he feels she is taking over his life. He has banished her to her own home out of the city. 'You can only stay one night at a time,' he told her before she left for the train. Now he is alone again for much of the day and night. He receives disability benefits in full and has a further grant from a charity (The Independent Living Fund) to enable him to live independently for the remainder of his life. Social services provide input for 7½ hours per week.

He said, 'The home care service should prioritize their work. In the past when I was well they would visit when I didn't really need them. There must be others who don't really need them now. If they stopped going to them they could give me more of the help I need now.'

Although David has had pneumonia and is recovering from tuberculosis, he was well enough to make the journey to my office. He was worrying about his death and, in particular, his funeral. 'I don't want one of those pauper's jobs for my funeral,' he said. 'It will cost quite a lot and I want to start saving for it. How shall I go about it?' I referred him to Immunity, a charity offering legal assistance to people with HIV and AIDS.

A man who I had been assisting during the past four months telephoned me. I had first known him at a time when he was homeless and had not long been out of hospital following a bout of pneumocystis carinii pneumonia (PCP). At that time, he had been living in a one-bedroom flat which he rented from a housing association. He needed a great deal of practical help. I assisted him with applications for a taxi card, a travel permit, a telephone, some grants for decorations, a bed, a fridge/freezer, a cooker and a washer/drier. Today he telephoned me wanting a television. I paused to think a little. If this were me, then not only may I want a television but I may want absolutely anything that I could get. For example, if I wanted an exotic holiday I would need help with travel. Perhaps some of this wanting may be a search for compensation for the price I was having to pay for living with this virus. Put in this context, what, if anything, could be deemed to be unreasonable? What, if anything, could compensate? How might these things equate with what can be provided?

Listening to people with HIV talk about their lives will very often highlight the need for material things. This can range from basic housing needs and assistance with respite care to the provision of cookers and other household goods such as televisions. It is useful in our work with people with HIV/AIDS to remember that 'respite' refers to a break in a convalescent environment in the broadest sense. In the mind of the professional, this might suggest a week in a hospice. In the mind of the person with HIV/AIDS, it may suggest a week by the sea or a weekend in Paris.

The extent to which it is part of the social work role to respond to these material requests can be a controversial question. Recently, I spoke to a director of a social services department who expressed the view that welfare rights work should be *arranged* by social workers rather than *provided* by them. In a similar manner, if someone needed counselling, social workers would arrange such a service rather than provide it. Already in some areas of Britain this definition of the social worker's role has been translated into practice. Changes in thinking about social work sometimes seem to be happening so fast that it is not surprising that social workers themselves have a lack of clarity about their role.

Work with people with HIV and AIDS is a relatively new area for social workers. Because of this area's short history it is arguably easier to target this work as a place to pilot new ways of working. Alongside this, we can see ways in which equal opportunities have made an impact on social work. One example can be seen in social work education. Training programmes that have been developed in the area of HIV education include courses on 'Ethnic communities and HIV', 'Women and HIV', 'People with learning difficulties and HIV', etc.

For a short time, I changed jobs to become a full-time trainer in HIV and AIDS awareness in a social services department. As an educator, I was forced to think about some of the theoretical issues relating to social work with people with HIV and AIDS. I found many social workers were still very concerned about the possibility of contracting HIV from clients with the virus. Far fewer appeared to be concerned about their own unsafe sexual activity in their personal lives. Even fewer had given any real thought to their roles as social workers. Often they would tell me they worked with children, the elderly, people with learning difficulties, etc. but that they did not work with people with HIV. It was amazing to me that so many had not realized that HIV was an issue for any of the client-groups within the social services – there are children with AIDS, elderly people with AIDS, people with learning difficulties with AIDS.

To educate social workers in the area of HIV/AIDS I would have to think carefully about the roles of social workers and the contributions that they could make. I would also need to think carefully about the statutory responsibilities that they face regarding children. These responsibilities are not changed by HIV/AIDS. As social workers in child care begin to encounter HIV in their work, the debate comes alive.

What I was beginning to learn now was that my past role as a fostering social worker had far more relevance than I had perhaps first realized. It would stand me in very good stead if I were to become involved in child care work where HIV had become an issue. Indeed, when I was finally asked for advice in relation to such a case, it was my background in child care which proved to be most valuable. It was now that I began to realize that the skills social workers needed to work with people with HIV/AIDS were skills that they would have developed in their work with other groups of people. Knowledge about medical aspects of HIV/AIDS would be relatively easy to acquire whereas skills in child care social work are developed through extensive practice under close supervision.

Social workers have for many years provided services to people with disabilities and to those faced with illness and death. Non-specialist workers in my office know that HIV can affect anyone, for example: if a woman has HIV, it doesn't mean she has used drugs or is black. Workers in my office know this, not because they have been told or because they have been on training events, but because they work with people with HIV who do not fit the stereotypes of people with HIV/AIDS that we read about in tabloid press. They have learned that many of the skills they have developed in their work with illness and disability are indeed transferable.

For example, a colleague of mine had been working with a woman with advanced HIV disease. At the point of referral, the woman had just been discharged from hospital and a request from the ward staff had been received to provide assistance with community care. At the point of initial assessment, there were a large number of professionals and volunteers involved, including the hospital discharge team, the community domiciliary care team, volunteers, the community liaison nurse and district nurses. At first sight it seemed that there may not have been a role left for the social worker. The competing pressure of other work and referrals could perhaps have tempted the team to give a low priority for this referral on the grounds that there were so many others involved. Such a course of action would have devalued the social work contribution and failed to have recognized the statutory responsibilities of social workers in local authorities, that is, legislation relating to mental health, children and community care.

Through the course of her visits, my colleague found her client wasting and becoming increasingly confused; her periods of lucidity became less frequent as each day passed. The doctors and nurses had another language to describe her condition but it seemed futile to persist in referring to manuals and books which might help decipher medical codes – by now it was clear that she was dying. My colleague was not sure what she was doing on her visits to her client. At the end of each visit she would arrange a further visit which seemed always too far away for her client, who would have liked, at this stage, a visit each day. I suggested to her that just being there might be enough and that at times like this we have to let go of the tangible things that we do. Perhaps short visits are best. Anything needing to be said can be said in minutes rather than hours. Listening, and I mean really listening, is what social workers can do at this point. If we feel that by just listening we are not doing anything, we could question ourselves about our need to 'do'. Is it that we need to do something to make **ourselves** feel better? At times of death we can often see that distress is not located in the dying but in those around them.

In my office we laugh and we joke. We do this especially when we are working with the dying. We think that laughter and humour can be a way of coping with our own distress. Some places of work have developed structured support systems for workers. Often this can be in groups with a facilitator. Some years ago I had worked in a multidisciplinary team in a psychiatric unit which adopted such a strategy. Each week we would attend a staff group. An assumption was made that the purpose of this group was to promote good working relationships and to create a feeling of support for each worker. In fact, quite the opposite occurred. Tension between workers grew. The staff team became very inward-looking. Morale and productivity fell while sickness levels rose and no one ever had any fun at work any more. Workers in the team became angry and felt that they were not valued and recognized. Formerly, I had worked in a therapeutic community in a psychiatric hospital where I had witnessed a more positive process. In any event, the question of support of social workers may be a key issue to address given the particular issues relating to their ever-changing (and poorly defined) role.

I try to organize my work with people with HIV/AIDS in such a way that it allows for the unpredictability that is so common with this condition. Most of my work is not organized on an appointment basis. I try to see people when they have a need to see me. This means that I have to try to arrange my time so that it gives me the flexibility to respond at short notice. This is not always easy and the danger is that my work could become chaotic. Conversely, operating an appointment system would mean that I had less ability to respond to the unpredictable. However, I try to see my clients in the late morning or afternoon and to be aware of their need for rest. It's important to be sensitive about when it's convenient to visit.

While many people with HIV/AIDS remain well, a sudden change in health can catapult someone from complete self-reliance to high dependence in only a matter of days. Last week a person who told me about an emotional roller-coaster of feelings after a diagnosis of HIV could this week need me to arrange appropriate care and raise money to buy a washing machine to make such care possible. At these times we, as social workers, can deploy our skills in assisting in the tangible and practical ways which can contribute considerably to the quality of someone's life. We should advocate for good housing and adequate finance which are the essential building blocks of a supportive environment for people with HIV/AIDS.

Our role in mobilizing the essentials of community care could be a key factor in making it possible for those with HIV/AIDS to retain a sense of choice and freedom to make decisions. In the process of offering such assistance, we should be mindful of our listening skills so that those using our services may feel that we are someone that they can talk to should they wish.

A man had agreed to tell me when the time of his dying had arrived. I knew that I would have to listen well when I was to hear him tell me this. I was thankful that skills that I had learned while working in mental health settings, with children and with drug-users were indeed transferable and usable in this situation.

Any work that I did with people with HIV/AIDS could be built on the skills that I had learnt in other areas of social work. One day, I visited him at a hospice after receiving a request via the nurses to help him sort out a minor financial problem. When I arrived, he told me that he wanted to go home. 'We will support you in this aim in the best way we can,' I said, 'What was it you needed me to do about your money?' 'Oh, nothing,' he said, 'It's not going to be long now.' I would perhaps see him once more when we had managed to get him home to die. First, my task was to advocate for his discharge from the hospice, and to identify and mobilize the help and support he would need in order to make his wish possible. To check that I understood him correctly I had asked him if the 'bottom line' was that he would need round-the-clock care and attendance. 'Oh, no,' he said, 'The bottom line is that I don't want to die.'

CONCLUDING REMARKS

As social workers we are not alone in our work with people with HIV/AIDS and we do not have a monopoly on any support, counselling or practical help that may be relevant. Those with HIV/AIDS will choose their own counsellors, helpers and people they wish to talk with about the issues that they face in their lives. They will choose who they wish to talk to about living and dying with AIDS. The social worker may be well-placed to respond to such a cocktail of different social needs. If we have been chosen to perform such a role, then we should attempt to perform it with good grace and to the best of our ability. When others have been chosen, we should find ways to support them.

We should remember that HIV is an issue for all users of our services and that the label of HIV/AIDS may be just one of many others – parent, daughter, teacher, son, doctor, social worker, neighbour, colleague, girlfriend, boyfriend, sexual partner, to name but a few. HIV/AIDS affects the communities in which we live as well as the places in which we work. We should do what we can to improve the quality of the lives of people with HIV/AIDS and remember that it is most often they who are best placed to tell us how to do this.

7

A service user's perspective

Ivor Lyford

INTRODUCTION

Let me introduce myself and put the following chapter into context. I am a 32-year-old gay man with AIDS and live with my partner in London. Many of the things I talk about will be familiar to people with HIV/AIDS, such as prejudice and discrimination. Other subjects, like what services or help is available locally, will be unfamiliar. This obviously will depend largely on where you live and who you are.

Many in the developing world will be struggling with the economic devastation that HIV disease has caused, so that when I talk about therapies such as massage later, it can seem an absurd luxury to those living in non-affluent countries who are worried about basic necessities such as clean water, nutritious food, and medical supplies. However, I wish to write about my experience of living with the virus in a city in the developed world, with all its advantages and point out some of the things that could be improved. These may not be only material things. I believe that there is more commonality in the larger body of people worldwide infected with the virus, than there is difference. I do however acknowledge the difference according to who you are. I cannot pretend to know what added issues will affect a woman with AIDS, a haemophiliac child, a drug-user, a heterosexual man, let along someone from another country with its own special circumstances. However, I can tell my story, which is that of a gay, middle-class Asian man living in contemporary London with a diagnosis of AIDS.

To be told you are HIV positive or have AIDS, whoever you are, is a crushing and devastating event in one's life. The sheer weight of feelings overwhelms you to begin with: can they (the staff) be wrong? Surely they don't mean me; have they got the right number or result? These feelings melt into terrific fears. There is fear of death, fear of disability, fear of pain, fear of disfigurement, fear of the unknown. There is also anxiety and great uncertainty. Questions such as, 'How long have I got? Who gave it to me? Who have I given it to? Who will I tell? (parents, partner, children, work colleagues), Can I go on working and for how long? What infections and cancers will I get and how will this affect me?'

Such questions preoccupy one's thoughts continually at first so that often one is in a paralysing emotional state and not able to consider the ordinary things in life. Friends of mine with the virus have felt many differing things: some felt anger and rage, others tremendous sadness and grief. Some felt hopelessness and had suicidal thoughts, others experienced a rage to live and a new spiritual hope. Some were depressed and had poor self-esteem, others found a revalued image and a new network of friends and support. Added on to this are our own extra doses of individual concerns depending who we are. My own concerns, the added discrimination and prejudice against my sexuality and my colour since I am a black, gay man.

People's overt or covert disgust around homosexuality have produced some of the most hurtful things I've heard. 'I don't want to work around queers with AIDS. They deserve it.' This attitude, though extreme, is present in some workers that I've met, though of course they wouldn't say it to me personally. Such phrases are overheard, but even small degrees of this attitude will be picked up by a sensitive person.

This is not to say workers should spend thousands of pounds on terminology-sensitivity training or ideological debates around HIV/AIDS. The purpose of the debate is to assist in creating an 'AIDS-educated environment'. I heard this phrase for the first time at York University in the early 1990s, when Jonathan Grimshaw (of Body Positive and Landmark) spoke at a conference on the neuropsychiatric aspects of HIV. Certainly from my point of view, what is practical and what addresses my needs at any one time is tangible help, here and now for me. Many people with AIDS want and need services quickly. Tomorrow may be too late, taking into account the appalling prognosis. Therefore I have a sense of urgency about things which workers in the field sometimes do not share (unless they live with someone with the virus or have the virus themselves).

Broadly speaking, from a service user perspective it is easy to divide the care providers into three areas: the voluntary agencies, the medical services and local government services, e.g., housing and social services. From my diagnosis as HIV positive to the present day (living with AIDS now for 4½ years), I've dipped in and out of many services as my needs have changed with time. Below, I talk about some events chronologically and mention my needs at those times, how I was helped and my view of the services. I shall also try to say how it could have been better in an ideal world.

THE EARLY PHASE

When I was first diagnosed in 1985 it was after a worrying period when I found I had enlarged lymph nodes in my neck. The service I used was my local sexually-transmitted disease clinic (now called the genito-urinary medicine clinic), and I spoke to the consultant physician who had seen me on a few occasions prior to this. I needed reassurance and to know what was going on.

Retrospectively, I think I should have had pre-test counselling to take time to understand the implications of an HIV test result. Such counselling services were in their infancy in the United Kingdom at that time. I did not receive the service. The result of the HIV test was positive. Post-test counselling would have given me the opportunity to talk through the overwhelming feelings that I described earlier. The doctor told me very little. I could only take in very little information after the shocking news, but even just the questions I asked should have been answered as openly and honestly as possible. The useful point here is that long information-giving sessions at this time are inappropriate – make another appointment later.

THE SYMPTOMATIC PHASE

The next two years were uneventful, and I quietly went into a kind of denial. I was sure I would not fall sick. I was immortal and special. So, I used no other services and contacted no self-help groups or agencies. I did not want to know or be associated with anything to do with HIV and AIDS. However in 1987, I was admitted to hospital with disseminated tuberculosis of my lymph nodes and lung tuberculosis. Initially, I was in a state of extreme panic because I thought that I had a lymphoma. I was put in a side room and made to feel like a leper by the staff. Nurses came in looking worried; my food tray was gingerly handled. I felt awkward about being gay because I felt this institution knew nothing about the sorts of friends I kept, my partner or my social life.

Under local anaesthetic, I had a surgical procedure. The anaesthetist and surgeon were cold and efficient. This I did not mind. My biopsy was sent to the laboratory and the staff there panicked and couldn't deal with it properly. Hence, I had to have a second unnecessary operation due to a mistake possibly due to ignorance and prejudice, possibly due to inefficiency or just bad luck. I was furious. However, when you feel ill, you don't want to complain or write letters. You want the job done quickly – and then you want to get out.

I really would have appreciated a little more normal chatter with the nurses. I know they're busy but just a little time to reassure would have been helpful. Secondly I would have benefited from the offer of a social worker since I was off work and in need of benefits advice, advocacy around financial matters and practical help. The offer of a spiritual person, such as a priest in my case, was also something I needed since I felt death was so close all the time. I suppose I could call myself a lapsed Catholic, but at this time religion reared its head again for me.

An improvement in the hospital food would have helped – perhaps foods appropriate to other cultures could have been included. A dietitian would have helped in devising a programme or diet to boost my weight and protein intake and to help reduce my diarrhoea.

This admission precipitated a huge spiritual and emotional crisis. I felt unable to manage my council flat on my own. My mum came to look after me for one month. In retrospect I could have been offered help with home care tasks until my strength had returned. This would have left my mum the choice of returning to her work and not taking dependency leave. I needed help with shopping, cleaning the flat, and preparing lunch and dinner. I believe there are now specialist HIV/AIDS home care teams. The importance is round-the-clock service, especially in the evening. Possibly a peripatetic care worker living in would be a good idea.

I had all the 'home help' type services from a relative. Others aren't so lucky. My mum had accepted my homosexuality since the time I had 'come out' to her. My father had long died. Many gay men have not told their parents about their homosexuality and fear rejection. Some *are* rejected. Their families are hearing two things that are really difficult. First that their son is gay; then, that he has AIDS and may die soon. Even if sexuality is not an issue, there will certainly be questions about how the virus was contracted, which may bring up a whole host of things not talked about before.

Upon being discharged to my flat, I convalesced with my mum's help. If I had not had her help, a respite facility such as is available locally could have been arranged or at least offered. However, recommending a place with a religious background like a traditional hospice is fraught with areas of concern. I would immediately think: What will their attitude to my homosexuality be? Would they try to convert me? Would they welcome my partner staying? Would they pity and patronize me, and treat me as a victim of 'God's wrath'?

Such anxieties have to be contradicted by caring, unprejudiced, sensitive and loving service. The church has a role here – as Kubler-Ross believes. AIDS poses the ultimate challenge to us all in that people with AIDS are not 'the judged' but each and every one of us will be judged by our response to this epidemic.

Back to the practicalities: My bed sheets were being washed almost daily because of drenching night sweats soaking them every night. My bath lacked rails and handles to help me emerge from it, and similarly the toilet lacked the same. I was weak, debilitated, unmotivated and chronically depressed. A cheery visit by an optimistic occupational therapist (albeit a stereotyped picture that I paint!) would have been both practical and beneficial to the spirits.

Can I make a few points here about home visits and me? Try not to look frightened. People who fear going into the houses of people with HIV/AIDS are not helping me feel good about myself. So please don't load me with your fears and anxieties at a time when I am sick and least able to cope. Secondly, a brightness of affect helps – a smile, a happy demeanour. If I'm miserable, it may cheer me up a little. If I remain miserable, nothing is lost.

Thirdly, humour is a healer. I believe it helps my immune system. So, a well-timed laugh and a joke may be more of a service than an efficient, nervous, anxious interview, then a scurry for the door, refusing any offer of food or drink in case of contamination, and an audible sigh of relief when the front door thuds!

A patient convalescing from an opportunistic infection goes through a range of emotions. My overwhelming feelings were of isolation and loneliness. Initially, I approached the Terrence Higgins Trust, because of spiritual reasons, in that I wanted to make contact with someone who understood my concerns in that area. It could equally have been a 'buddy' that I wanted, and indeed I was offered one following a visit by the buddy coordinator. My buddy's assumption was that I was in such an awful situation as he perceived it, that he could not befriend me without special skills and a training in how to deal with people with AIDS. At first, I did not make it clear enough that providing for the practical tasks such as cooking a lunch, or mopping the kitchen floor would have made me feel better rather than an in-depth counselling session. People with a life-threatening condition do not necessarily need to 'talk it through' continually, or require counselling in the psychiatric sense. This already is the beginning of a process of treating people as patients, which is more comfortable and safe for those involved, rather than seeing the person as a human being facing certain challenges.

I will just mention here that while I had tuberculosis in my old flat, I decided to take up another service provided by the Terrence Higgins Trust called 'helper cells'. These are volunteers who perform practical tasks, and though I needed help with redecorating the flat, I picked up the phone with some trepidation. The man who came around was fine, and the painting was done. But I was left feeling that he needed support and someone to talk to more than I did. This is fine if it is mutually beneficial, but so often I hear the same story from people with AIDS: they feel they have to support the helper. Sometimes this will make you feel that it is easier to do it yourself if you possibly can, or wait until you're better.

I handle the dilemma of wanting care at appropriate times, and not wanting the 'patient' role which disempowers me, by ensuring that at all times I am not being made into an object by others, that I am not being patronized, and by insisting that my voice is heard and not marginalized. This, as you can imagine, needs constancy and strength. Sometimes, when I look dreadful, feel ill, and read horrific things written about AIDS in the media, my resolve can falter. That's when I need a friend, a chat and a boost.

I did join a group at the Terrence Higgins Trust, which helped me not feel so freakish and lonely. Of course it is very difficult sometimes because people fall ill and die in the life of a group. I wonder if I would be next. I experienced what is sometimes known as 'survivor guilt' – I had no idea why I was still living while others had died. The guilt of the survivor is very difficult to deal with at times. The Terrence Higgins Trust also gave welfare rights advice. Since I was not working now, this was a very practical intervention. I felt poor suddenly, unable to pay my telephone bill, or sort out some debts that I'd incurred. In retrospect, it might have been useful if the Terrence Higgins Trust worker had suggested seeing a social worker, either from the hospital I was attending, or in the borough I lived in, to be an advocate for me. Perhaps an application could have been made to a charity to help with a one-off payment to British Telecom. Meanwhile, a kind friend helped me. If not, I would have to deal with feelings of shame and guilt, and perhaps ask for charitable help from an agency. There is a much-discussed topic among the cognoscenti (that is, people with the virus and their allies) that money donated to AIDS charities does not often get right down the chain to relieve directly the distress of people with HIV/AIDS. There is so much red tape that a lot of the money ends up spent on people called 'AIDS careerists' or 'AIDS parasites'. This, no doubt, is a problem that is neither new nor exclusive to the world of HIV disease. My answer is simple: place the needs of the person with HIV/AIDS foremost, and that will be a good guide. Square it with your own conscience.

HOUSING

My gay lover and I now needed to think seriously about where we were living. It was a first-floor council flat, with stairs to manage, and I was feeling vulnerable on several accounts. First, I had been used to abuse about being gay, which sometimes made me feel very unsafe on the estate. However, if anyone suspected I now had AIDS, I feared what would happen, as has happened to some I know: dog excrement and lit newspapers put through the letter box, abuse scrawled on the front door.

I applied for a transfer to more suitable accommodation. My argument was that if my health deteriorated any more (which is very likely), I would need ground-floor accommodation or accommodation suitable for wheelchair users. I needed to be near my treatment centre, which was several miles away and in a different borough. I wished to be nearer my support network, my lover's family and to be in a 'safe' area.

This brings up the issue of confidentiality. I had been advised that if I did disclose my predicament to the local borough housing department, it would help me tremendously. I could then be classified vulnerable on medical grounds, and also on social grounds due to gay harassment. I thought long and hard and made an appointment with my housing officer at the town hall (not my estate manager, since I did not wish him to know about my HIV status). I told the housing officer that what I was about to say was strictly confidential and that no documentation should link my name and address with HIV or AIDS. 'A1 Medical Priorities' labels can be given without mentioning AIDS; for instance, I wished tuberculosis to be used as the reason for being given medical priority.

My lover and I anxiously waited three months. I decided that I needed further support to quicken things up and contacted my local ward councillor. Putting it bluntly, I said I did not wish to die waiting for a housing transfer. This is a reality when dealing with agencies such as local councils, whose waiting lists are often longer than the prognosis of life after an AIDS diagnosis. I needed to impress the urgency again here, and I chose to disclose to certain key people who I hoped would assist me. Other people in my situation sometimes do not wish to say they have HIV and AIDS. Of course that is their privilege to do so, but in times of few resources, they may not be rehoused or it may take longer than they hoped.

I was referred to the London Area Mobility Scheme, by the housing manager. I wished to be nominated to a sympathetic housing association. Two weeks later, a housing association worker interviewed me about a possible property, adapted for the disabled. I was concerned that the housing association did not discriminate against lesbians and gay men. What would happen when I died? Would my partner be asked to leave the flat? Would they let him stay on for a while? Would they commit themselves to rehouse him? Often, joint tenancies give certain protection, but it's best to get good legal advice about this.

The Inland Revenue was hassling me over some outstanding tax that needed to be paid. I phoned them up and made an appointment to see a tax officer. She was very sympathetic to the fact that I was now chronically sick. However, I told her I had tuberculosis and not HIV. She asked me to make a reasonable proposal, in view of the fact I was on social security benefits, to repay the debt. My proposal, a monthly payment, was accepted and another weight was off my mind. I did continue to be hassled on a yearly basis however, to fill in tax forms. I contacted my social worker at the hospital I had been attending, to write to the Inland Revenue, because I wanted an advocate with some authority behind her.

After receiving an 'official' letter to explain the situation, I was bothered no further.

A SURGICAL EXPERIENCE

Another time my partner and I used a social worker was when we were far from home, on holiday in a remote part of England, and my appendix burst. After I was admitted as an emergency through casualty to intensive care, the medical team referred me to the surgical team, who took a long time to make a decision to operate. I suspected that the surgeon involved was HIV-phobic, and was trying to avoid operating on someone with 'tainted blood' with the remote possibility of the surgeon being infected by accidental inoculation. This was later confirmed to me by a junior doctor after the event. Such a dangerous action as delaying my operation because of personal fears could have, ironically, resulted in my death not from an HIV-related illness, but from peritonitis which is not directly HIV-related. I understand the surgeon's concerns, but I feel that, morally, the decision not to operate is unacceptable in a civilized, caring society. Why should I be penalized for letting the medical staff know in advance of my condition, when probably the surgeon is sometimes operating on patients who have not taken an HIV test, and are HIV positive, or those who know they are positive but choose not to disclose this?

Rather than just looking at this issue from the perspective of the uninfected possibly being exposed to HIV-infected material, we must question the risks to the person with HIV who has a weakened immune system. If it is assumed that everyone who is not tested is HIV negative, that is, therefore has 'safe' blood, and different, less efficient sterilizing and cleaning procedures are performed, might this not endanger people with HIV with weakened immune systems who need operations? What of the HIV status of the surgeon performing an operation? Is the patient or surgeon more or less at risk from the other? These questions need further exploration, but it helps if people can broaden their vision and see things from the perspective of the vulnerable person with HIV/AIDS. The same health and safety precautions should be taken for every person, whether or not it is known that the person is HIV positive. That way, safety is ensured.

There should not be a development of apartheid, where there is one set of rules for the untested, and another for the tested. People with AIDS face enough social, legal, cultural and personal discrimination all the time, without the medical establishment joining in as well.

My partner and I felt we needed a social worker at this point to help us through it all. The social worker had never worked with people with AIDS before and said so. However, her already acquired skills meant that my partner was supported, and I had someone advocating for me whilst I was an in-patient in a tiny rural cottage hospital.

Complementary therapies do not replace the medical treatment one receives (although some people choose to do this), but can be done in addition to them. There are a whole host of therapies ranging from reflexology and aromatherapy to meditation and yoga. Many HIV organizations provide subsidized, nutritious and delicious lunches, and this service acts as a drop-in centre where people can meet in a natural social setting which can help if one is feeling isolated and lonely. However, it may also be depressing to hear some people's tales, and to see how people look. It can be a reminder that one might end up with the same ailments.

I wish now to address the issue of 'significant others' in the lives of people with AIDS. Do think of the infected person as surrounded by different people affected by HIV. For instance, I have already mentioned my mum. Not everyone tells their parents for a start. However, I would not be presumptuous enough to say I knew what my mum went through during the last six years. She had her own special needs, her need for support, the problem of who to tell, coping with feelings of shame and guilt, etc. The Terrence Higgins Trust and London Lighthouse run a 'Family Support Group' which meets once a month. It's usually held at the weekends to enable people living outside London to attend, especially if they're working. My mum attended and I think she told me she found the meetings very good in the beginning. She talked to other mothers and has retained some friends from this group. She went for about one year, then no longer felt the need to continue. She presently does volunteer work at the local Body Positive helpline.

My lover has the choice of a 'gay men's group' at the London Lighthouse, or a 'partner's group' of those with the virus. I say choice because he chooses not to go at present. However it is good to know what is available, including bereavement counselling services. I feel that specialist gay services are sometimes very helpful, because they are more able to talk about sensitive issues such as gay sex. In London, a number of diverse projects do exist which provide counselling and training for gay people, heterosexual individuals and mixed groups. Some of the projects are specialist, others generic.

MEDICAL CARE

My clinic doctor sees me roughly once a month for regular checkups. When I was HIV positive and asymptomatic it was every 3–6 months. As the condition progresses I expect I will be reviewed at shorter and shorter intervals.

I personally find going to the clinic a stressful experience. The agonizing wait before seeing the doctor and the inevitable questions occur time and time again. Have my T-cells dropped? Will my blood tests from the last visit show any problems such as anaemia? Will I need a transfusion? Will I need to stop a particular medication or start a new one? What will the side-effects be? Am I ill, despite feeling well?

The last question is an important one. Even if absolutely fine, a hospital visit can precipitate much anxiety about my health. Am I then a hypochondriac? No, I think all such anxiety is understandable. Sometimes, the doctors and nurses (even specialist HIV doctors and nurses) forget this.

Having mentioned the long wait, which can be frustrating and painful, I regularly meet others in the waiting area. It can be quite a game working out if people are HIV positive or not, but if it is a specialist waiting area, this question is already answered: Yes (by definition)! Shifty glances at each other can eventually melt into small friendly chats.

I have found a specialist HIV receptionist to be a great bonus. He or she may reassure you, make you laugh and generally normalize the situation. Also, a cup of coffee while waiting eases the frustration.

I see a consultant in genito-urinary medicine. We have known each other now for eight years and our relationship is an important one as it is built on trust, honesty and mutual respect. Many people change their physician at times of deteriorating health or they become angry at them for various reasons. I think this is great. If one is not happy with one's doctor, sort it out or change doctors. A San Francisco cohort of gay men with AIDS living longer than five years (that is, long-term survivors), all had challenging relationships with the medical establishment, sacking medical personnel from their care when they thought fit.

After two years, due to a clash of personalities I managed to change my HIV specialist nurse. Initially I was concerned that this would sour all my other relationships with the staff, but I need not have worried. I have found that the benefits outweigh the disadvantages. My relationship with the new nurse is good. Wearing gloves, she takes my blood, weighs me, chats, lets me help myself to condoms, needles and syringes; then I leave with a huge plastic bag full of medications for the month ahead. I keep the equipment for aerosolized pentamidine (pneumocystis carinii pneumonia prophylaxis) at home, since I prefer to do this myself in the comfort of my own home. Other friends say they prefer to go to the clinic and let the nurse set it up. It takes about one hour in all (every two weeks in my case), and is a hassle. If I forget to do it, I feel guilty and vulnerable.

A specialist HIV pharmacist sat in at every regular visit. This helped in that I could ask about the various therapies I was taking, and discuss the side-effects with her. She was up-to-date on all the experimental and trial drugs, and she would bring my monthly supply of DDI (an antiviral medication), plus my anti-tuberculosis medications with her, saving me an extra trip to the pharmacy department. When I stopped AZT (Zidovudine) and started DDI, she could tell me about some of the preliminary findings from the trials in the United States. This is an example of how I am very involved in my treatment, and really direct it myself with help from discussions, reading and medical monitoring.

I have seen the HIV dietitian once or twice, after my appendicitis admission, and since I lost weight. She advised on a weight-gain diet and gave me high-calorie supplements in the form of drinks. The drinks come in different flavours but taste sickly. She was able to reassure me, and encourage me not to worry about eating too much fat or sugar. Sometimes reducing sugar helps people with thrush in their mouths though I find it makes no difference. Live yoghurt also helps some people.

During a difficult time in my relationship with my partner, I did see a health adviser for a few sessions. The quality of 'counselling' I received was not impressive, but it was comforting to know they were there, and for reasons other than just pre- and post-test counselling.

The debate about having specialist workers in this field rests on whether indeed specialists are more up-to-date with information in a rapidly changing area of research. I have received excellent treatment from generic workers as well; my experience is that workers who have had some HIV training are in some ways better prepared than untrained workers. It is infuriating to deal with workers' anxieties about 'catching it' when I know the likelihood is almost nil. It is grossly insensitive and insulting to people with HIV/AIDS to have workers with transmission fears, because this feeds into our negative feelings of being dirty, untouchable and unattractive. These feelings should be contradicted with touch, care and concern, and not with gloves, masks and space suits.

Many people with HIV know more than health care workers because they read the medical press and complementary medicine articles and journals. This should not make the worker feel disempowered I hope. If workers retreat behind a stance of 'I know it all' or 'I know better than you', problems arise, but an educated discussion of the issues can be beneficial to both parties. This, of course, challenges the notion of the patient as a passive recipient of services and treatments, which may make certain workers uncomfortable and threatened. True health care is a partnership, an open dialogue, not a prescription of laws and rules.

GENERAL PRACTITIONERS AND HIV

I made a decision to let the clinic tell my general practitioner (GP) about my HIV quite a long time after my diagnosis. Up to that point I was worried that GPs knew very little about the disease. Now that GPs have their own budgets, they might not want me on their list because I would be an expensive patient. Some GPs have personal prejudices against gay men, as well as being prejudiced against black people. In terms of insurance companies, I knew my GP would not lie for me and would reveal my diagnosis of AIDS if asked. However, when I moved area, I registered with a new GP who now knows I have AIDS. She is very good and supportive and when she needs to reveal my diagnosis to a third party, she rings me first to ask my permission. This gives me back the control of who I wish to know about my diagnosis.

I decided to be open about my HIV status with my new GP because I thought it might be easier if I needed further services, e.g., home care, district nurse, etc. (of course, these services can be obtained without the help of a GP). Some people with HIV/AIDS do not want to tell their GP in case the GP tells the rest of the family (which would be a breach of confidentiality, but nevertheless can happen). Others do not tell their GP because they get all their care wholly from genito-urinary clinics and hospitals.

Because the GP is very close and does home visits, I find I can go with my minor ailments such as sore throats, verrucas, inoculations and boils; and she is very vigilant about the HIV side of things. She signs my sick notes, and we meet roughly four times a year. She recently phoned up the Department of Social Security to put off a medical examination which was an extra unnecessary hassle for me. She is not particularly up-to-date on HIV matters, but she remains a good, solid, caring doctor whom I would like to be involved with my terminal care at home when the time comes.

TRANSPORT

Below, I mention three local government schemes that people with AIDS (and possibly HIV symptomatics) can be entitled.

- A free Travel Pass – In my area this is the London Regional Transport Travel Card applied for through a social work assistant in my borough. It allows free travel on buses and tubes.
- The Orange Badge Scheme for Parking – This allows a person with a disability to park in certain areas where others would not be allowed to. I have used my mobility allowance to join Motability, where a car can be leased for three years including all servicing and repair costs. Additional benefits include cheaper insurance and possible road tax exemption.
- Taxicard Scheme – This allows, at vastly reduced prices, a journey by taxi, although there is a limit which is fare-dependent. This scheme varies slightly from borough to borough within London.

Travelling, and particularly driving my car, has maintained my independence tremendously. Even if it comes to a point where I cannot drive for medical reasons, my partner can then drive me as a named driver on the insurance.

RACE AND CULTURE

Finally, I would like to put the issue of race and culture on the agenda. Many cultures have taboos around homosexuality, and so it would seem that black gay people do not exist. Or so many people think. Actually, I do exist!

I face racism in the services I receive in a mild way. It is institutionalized into a system that sees only white British needs in general. While, in a multi-racial society like modern-day Britain, one cannot cater for every cultural difference and be sensitive to every ethnic minority, the service provider can start by at least thinking about ethnicity.

People from my part of the world were colonized by Europeans. We still have internalized feelings of inferiority, and it is harder to be assertive in a society that views us as 'native', or 'stupid' or even 'criminal'. AIDS can compound these feelings, especially if there are additional language difficulties.

It can help to have someone from one's own part of the world around. Workers should be aware of some of the difficulties ethnic minorities have in accessing services and how these services could be more sensitive to cultural difference. Remember, HIV affects all countries of the world.

No one yet knows the origins of HIV for certain. All theories reflect a particular position, or prejudice. The virus does not discriminate nor does it know if you are black or white, gay or straight, male or female, adult or child. It is people who discriminate and hold prejudice.

No single group of people is to blame.

CONCLUDING REMARKS

I suppose if I was asked what were the big contributions to the quality of my life post-diagnosis it would be (in no order of merit) establishing my housing; receiving high-quality medical care; reorganizing my finances so that I no longer existed on £30 weekly income support, and, finally, eating, sleeping and keeping well.

Love is so obvious that I almost don't mention it. I feel so loved by my partner, my family, and some friends that if I died tomorrow I would still consider myself lucky and privileged to have had such gifts.

A purpose to each day is important. This can be anything, even if it is appreciating the beauty of a sunset, or a good laugh with a friend, or looking forward to a treat like a meal out.

Getting rid of negative influences helps too. This may involve dropping a few false friends and relationships, sacking people, not doing things I hate because I think I ought to, or simply not being too critical of oneself.

Like most people, I tend to be better physically and emotionally after holidays – I feel it is to do with reducing stress. I wish I could prescribe long stress-free holidays to those who need them, with a secure, safe and loving home to come home to.

Some sort of hope is important, and this is not necessarily the spiritual hope that organized religion talks of. However, the spiritual dimension to my life has taken on a new meaning.

Lastly, I retain a sense of pride and dignity in who I am. Despite the epidemic of ignorance, discrimination and prejudice I know I deserve care, treatment and respect. I shall continue to demand basic human rights for those people living with HIV/AIDS, and those not so fortunate as myself.

Do not merely think of 'patients', 'clients', 'service users' with HIV/AIDS. They may yet turn out to be your 'teachers' if you listen well enough.

8

Multidisciplinary working

Louise Cusack and Surinder Singh

INTRODUCTION

This chapter is designed to illustrate the benefits of a multidisciplinary approach to the care of a particular patient with HIV infection. The case example highlights a man (A.S.) with HIV infection who developed a sudden onset illness which left him profoundly disabled. His rehabilitation and the challenges he presented form the focus of the chapter.

Uncommon though it is, sometimes such a serious disabling condition signals a slow and gradual deterioration in health. Whether this is because of HIV infection or the nature of the superimposed condition is beyond the remit of the chapter. Nevertheless in the case of A.S. he did become irretrievably ill approximately one year after the acute episode.

This latter phase of his illness presented new problems for not only himself but also his carers and the professionals looking after him. In other words, his requirements had changed but those caring for him could still meet his needs, although in a different way. How this was achieved is explained later in the chapter as the aim of therapy changed from the curative to the palliative. A.S. finally died in the way he wanted to, in a chosen place and surrounded by those who cared for him.

The end of this chapter is marked by a description of the fundamental principles of palliative care. Caring for those with a 'terminal illness' is not unique to HIV infection or AIDS. Six important principles are described in this chapter which pave the way to providing good quality, effective and compassionate palliative care.

CASE HISTORY: A.S.

A.S. was a 49-year-old postman who was gay and had known he was HIV positive for the previous six months. At the time he thought his health had deteriorated and he admitted to being at risk many years ago. Approximately 24 hours prior to admission to an acute medical ward, A.S. complained of sudden onset of pain in both legs before collapsing at home. He was taken to hospital where examination revealed a marked weakness in all muscle groups below the waist, diminished reflexes and sphincter disturbance. There was also patchy sensory loss with impairment of joint position sense in both legs. A.S. had been rendered paraplegic almost overnight.

Despite extensive investigations including CT and MRI scans, no definitive diagnosis could be made. Although empirical treatment commenced, A.S.'s condition remained static.

A.S. lived alone in West London, in a second-floor flat, and he had no family. His parents were both deceased. He described himself as a private man with two or three very good close friends. Others knew him only superficially. He had returned to Britain in the last 18 months, after living in Spain for many years.

He realized that the paraplegia would most likely be permanent, although he was aware of the uncertainty of the diagnosis despite a welter of blood tests, X-rays and special scans. He was shocked and bewildered by these recent events in his life although he began to adjust remarkably quickly following his admission to hospital. Inevitably he did experience frustration and periods of depression following the initial shock, though this was tempered, in his view, by the fact that life up to now had been fairly good to him, especially in his relationships, wealth and overall life-style.

Functional ability

Weight-bearing and standing were very difficult and could only be managed with two people supporting his weight. However, his upper limbs were spared and he retained good function in both his arms. He was naturally right-handed.

A.S. did have fairly poor bladder function which developed

soon after admission to hospital. He was not able to urinate spontaneously and was subsequently catheterized. His bowels, previously never a bother to A.S., were also adversely affected by his condition. Initially his appetite was poor and he became quite constipated. This was relieved with glycerine suppositories and he was commenced on a regular bowel programme.

The various members of the clinical team worked very closely during this period, especially in providing ongoing support. A.S. was determined, at this early stage, to make decisions regarding his care at all times.

Principles of treatment

The overall goal was for A.S. to become wheelchair-independent. In addition, A.S. was determined to return to his own environment with the necessary support to lead a life of as high a quality as possible.

Initially therefore, a period of assessment was arranged whereby A.S.'s condition, 'problems', and psychological state were defined in terms of needs. These broad areas then gave rise to treatment goals which were aimed at maximizing existing abilities and skills.

Moreover, prevention of deformaties and pressure sores, and maintenance of skin care were important nursing care objectives. A.S. throughout this process was assisted to adjust to these new circumstances with the help of various professionals. A more formal counselling role was provided by the social worker on this occasion.

In addition, A.S. attended a support group which he found quite useful. Here a number of issues were discussed including general health, medications and treatment regimes. One aspect of this type of support was that it enabled A.S. to express his feelings in a group which shared their experiences.

Factors in considering therapy

Time

A.S.'s tolerance to rehabilitation was initially limited due to his condition. Thus, work in the 'rehabilitation gym' was initially very light, but increased gradually over days and weeks. Since other members of the team needed to see A.S., his individually-tailored programme was planned in close collaboration with other professionals such as the physiotherapist and the occupational therapist.

Format

Usually work with A.S. was carried out on a one-to-one basis, the one exception to this being the support group.

Resources

This point was evident when resettlement was considered. Adaptation to the flat along with specialized equipment needed funding, though in this case A.S. could meet some of the cost himself.

Setting

Although much of the rehabilitation work was carried out in hospital, the overall aim of returning to the community was not forgotten. The aim for A.S. was to resettle at home in a suitable supportive environment; this desire became stronger the longer he remained in hospital.

Rehabilitation phase

As mentioned previously, an early assessment did suggest that wheelchair-independence was a viable objective, thus a wheelchair with cushion was introduced. As a result, areas such as personal care, transferring to and from the wheelchair and activities of daily living were to be addressed as a first step in realizing the overall goal of returning home.

Personal care

Most of A.S.'s personal care was carried out in his wheelchair at the 'vanity-style' sink, i.e. hair, nail care, dental hygiene and shaving. He was highly motivated since he felt his appearance affected his overall feeling of well-being. Dressing was always managed on his bed, and after a while he became independent at this. A long-handled shoe-horn and an 'easy-reach' (lightweight, long-handled aluminium grasper) were invaluable. A.S. took to wearing tracksuits most of the time, on account of comfort. Bathing, in contrast, was more difficult and could only be completed with practical help and the use of a hoist.

Transfers

The basic task of positioning in both wheelchair and chair had to be taught prior to teaching about transfers. With the use of a 'sliding-board' he did manage this task well and independently.

Activities of daily living

Basic personal activities of daily living have been mentioned. Because of preservation of upper-limb function, activities such as preparing drinks, snacks and cooking were possible and indeed encouraged. Useful equipment like lightweight tin-openers and the microwave cooker were of immense value. A.S. also managed to use a lightweight iron, although a special wall-mounted ironing board was required.

Leisure time

A.S. realized he could not return to work. He did receive a small but regular social benefit on account of his condition. One idea of his was to utilize his knowledge of Spanish, and contribute to a newsletter for a local HIV support group for those from Southern Europe. Transport to the centre was arranged through volunteer drivers, and this became a regular fixture for him over the ensuing weeks.

Resettlement

It became clear that A.S.'s flat was unsuitable for a wheelchair and could not be adapted with ease. Fortunately, a housing association had a small number of flats for this level of disability. He was finally offered a ground-floor flat, which was wheelchair-accessible and had two bedrooms. A.S. did visit the proposed flat with the occupational therapist and social worker before accepting it. A number of adaptations were necessary including some fixtures and fittings. The flat was unfurnished. A comprehensive discharge plan was going to be necessary before A.S. was to return home.

Once A.S. had agreed to the new flat, various home visits were carried out to assist in the fitting of disability equipment and in the decoration of the flat. Funding was sought and contributions were obtained from charity sources for the fixtures and fittings.

The following were general considerations for A.S. in the new flat:

- Electric sockets were raised with the use of extensions.
- Electric light switches were lowered to waist height.
- All items of storage were arranged and placed conveniently in such a way that commonly-used items remained accessible at all times.
- Flooring had to be as uncluttered as possible to enable easy manoeuvring. In addition, advice was given as to the type of floor covering, i.e. vinyl or tiles being more appropriate than deep pile carpets.
- Windows were difficult to clean thus electric fans were placed in the bathroom and kitchen.

Prior to discharge

Almost the biggest challenge in attempting to discharge A.S. from hospital and return to the community was the co-ordination of services necessary to ensure this happened smoothly and with the minimum of disruption. The co-operation of statutory services was required with voluntary services, in addition to a small number of friends who were keen to participate in helping A.S.

A 'key worker' system was established so that the roles and responsibilities of community health care workers became clear, and his progress could be monitored. Prior to discharge, a series of afternoon visits, overnight stays and weekend leave visits from hospital were arranged to enable the package of care to be tried and tested. In a small number of areas, the plan was amended and modified for the final discharge.

Home in the community

A.S. resettled successfully at home despite the disabilities mentioned earlier. A.S. lived at his new home for approximately a year; during this time he was fairly happy.

Intermittently A.S. resented the set of restrictions which had adversely affected the quality of his life. He often talked about his travels in and around Spain and the various temporary jobs he had tried in the UK and in Europe. He particularly missed the warm climate of southern Europe, especially the short winter and the prolonged summer months.

One of the facts which greatly distressed A.S. was how fit he was in the past, in great contrast to his present condition.

Despite these losses A.S. was determined to continue living as best he could. He enjoyed tremendously the Spanish Support Group. The fact that he could translate newsletters for the group gave him a feeling of 'worth' which he appreciated. He also found it quite taxing, especially if there were deadlines to meet. A.S. did meet up with friends on a regular basis and travelled, although he did not manage to visit Spain again. A.S. continued to attend the HIV clinic for regular monitoring.

Summary of support services for A.S.

- *Home helps*:
  Visited daily each week. Laundry, cleaning, shopping, food preparation and cooking.
- *Meals on wheels*:
  Provided meals daily or when necessary.
- *Housing association support worker*:
  Support with housing, maintenance and benefits/bills with housing.

- *Transport service*:
  Transport to/from day centre, hospital appointments/visits.
- *Night sitting service/live-in help*:
  Regular help arranged for overnight stay or 'live-in help' for a few days.
- *Respite care*:
  Arranged with local hospice for weekend stays.
- *Spanish support group*:
  Met weekly for emotional/psychological support. Occasional outings planned.
- *Aromatherapist*:
  Visited weekly at home for one-to-one sessions.
- *2 x Spanish support groups*:
  Two to three evenings per week provided an opportunity to meet other people.
- *Friends*:
  Informal social visits, occasionally assisted with meals.
- *GP*:
  Oversaw medical matters and provided continuing support.
- *District nurse*:
  Visited regularly, to assist with bowel/bladder management, medication and ongoing support.
- *Terrence Higgins Trust buddy*:
  Outings, befriending.
- *Social worker*:
  Provided support assistance with benefits/income housing and co-ordinated services as key worker.
- *Counsellor*:
  Regular counselling on a one-to-one basis.
- *Community physiotherapy; community occupational therapy*:
  Maintained wheelchair mobility and regular review of activities of daily living skills.

Advanced disease phase

After nine months, A.S. developed a chest infection, over a weekend, and was admitted to hospital as an emergency. Following extensive investigations, pneumocystis carinii pneumonia was excluded and a course of intravenous antibiotics was completed in hospital. He was discharged home soon after.

Following another period at home A.S. was again admitted to hospital with shortness of breath and chest pain. Despite investigations, no diagnosis was made and another course of antibiotics seemed beneficial.

It became clear at this stage that A.S. was much weaker than previously and had continued to lose weight. Formal examination during this latter admission revealed upper limb weakness with wasting of most muscle groups and a degree of sensory loss. There was also evidence of limited short-term memory impairment, again of fairly recent origin. Repeated non-invasive investigations, such as CT scanning and MRI imaging, revealed no obvious opportunistic infections. Although further investigations could have been performed, most felt little could be gained. A.S. himself had felt for some time that all efforts should now be directed towards maximizing comfort and maintaining, where possible, quality of life. He expressed this during lucid periods to his close friends, nursing staff and to the junior doctors working on the ward.

He did appear to relate very well to a small number of nurses and explained to them why he felt attempts to prolong his life were now not appropriate. He was always calm and rational during these conversations, expressing the desire to face his inevitable mortality with forthright courage and dignity. He also sincerely hoped the clinical staff would continue to treat him well, with compassion and allow him a dignified death. He held no firm religious beliefs.

It became apparent that A.S. did not wish to return home. He had discussed this with various people, including a few friends, and had decided to opt for residential hospice care.

He was duly referred, assessed and admitted to a hospice unit for which he was grateful. Even during this transition period A.S. declined inexorably with increasing weight loss, continued weakness and deteriorating mental function.

Although on admission to the hospice unit he was aware of the new surroundings, his rapid decline continued unabated. One of the newer features of his symptoms was a diffuse, deep ache present throughout all limbs which was only partially relieved by oral medications. Small doses of oral morphine were given a trial with some improvement, the pain becoming less prominent. A.S. soon required a subcutaneous delivery system for the morphine since swallowing was increasingly difficult. A.S. died peacefully two days later surrounded by his few chosen friends.

PALLIATIVE CARE

A good working definition of Palliative Care is that which is required most when an individual in whom, following an accurate diagnosis, the advent of death is certain and not too far distant and for whom treatment has changed from the curative to the palliative.

This important area within HIV/AIDS treatment has generally been hitherto neglected despite the increasing numbers of individuals who succumb to the infection and its many complications. It is clear, however, that there is an increasing imperative to acknowledge the advanced stages of this chronic infection, deal with the painful processes surrounding death, and again maximize choice in an area where options are naturally constrained and restricted.

The important underlying principles of palliative care are not different from the principles which guide those caring for patients with widespread carcinoma, lymphomas or other life-threatening diseases. In Britain and in the West the hospice movement has been most vociferous in identifying the complex needs of those who have a 'terminal' illness. As a result, palliative care is one of the fastest growing specialities in medicine, with new units opening and many adopting a community approach. Areas of priority include research, education and training, and the wider issue of ethics. It should therefore be possible for the experience of the last 30 highly productive years to be transferred swiftly to those with chronic HIV infection and AIDS.

Many patients with HIV/AIDS do enter an advanced stage, where the skills of palliative carers would be most appropriate. If approached in the right manner, this would signify a greater emphasis on quality of life without necessarily refusing 'active treatment'. It is possible to care for patients in a way which provides for palliation without foregoing life-saving treatment.

These principles are highlighted below, tailored to HIV infection and AIDS.

Symptom control

An important facet of palliative care is controlling troublesome symptoms, be they the obvious such as pain, or the seemingly trivial like a dry mouth. Many of the troublesome symptoms can be alleviated, if not removed entirely. Pain, anorexia, nausea, insomnia and constipation figure highly in the symptoms most frequently reported. General high-quality nursing is a central feature in providing this type of care. It has been estimated (outside of the HIV-affected population) that pain affects about half of those receiving chemotherapy and three-quarters of those with advanced tumours. For those with advanced HIV infection and AIDS, these figures may well be similar since it is a multisystem disorder not unlike a disseminated tumour.

Multidisciplinary teamwork

Palliative care encompasses a special mix of skills which brings to patients interventions which alleviate symptoms, enhance the quality of life, restore some element of choice and ensure dignity at all times. Modern-day practice dictates that this can only occur with a multidisciplinary approach which includes clinicians, therapists, and carers as well as complementary therapists.

Hopefully, this combination should mean that, for someone affected, there is someone to talk with most of the time. Counselling and support services are available to assuage the fear and despair often experienced by those who are 'terminally ill' and are feeling isolated. Occupational therapists and physiotherapists may contribute specifically to pain-relieving measures as well as maintenance of function. A good social worker may be the only regular support for someone with HIV infection, and an acupuncturist may be the only therapist who can relieve the pain of a neuropathy.

Avoidance of inappropriate therapy

One of the much needed skills in this area is to distinguish between appropriate and inappropriate therapy at various stages in a patient's illness. On principle, this can only be decided by the person receiving care. However, those care workers involved will be influential in that decision, and of course, what may be appropriate this week may plainly not be so next week.

Support of carers and relatives

To be surrounded by loved ones, including friends, partner or family must fulfil an objective of care, especially if they can contribute to care and hence quality of life. Part of the care must be directed towards loved ones and it is only through these special relationships that the patient can be adequately supported. The relationship between staff and loved ones must take into account the pre-existing emotional bonds, their previous relationships and friends and perhaps the dynamics of the family. Since the average age of those affected by HIV infection is 35 years, this is no easy task. Spiritual care must be taken into account, sometimes initiated by the patient, sometimes only by a loved one or family member. A spiritual chaplain can help all in such trying times.

Continuity of care

For many with advanced HIV infection and AIDS, continuity of care signifies a vast array of care workers who all provide different aspects of care. For many patients, this is a most difficult area since no close relationship can be fostered and discontinuity may well ensue. In addition this array of carers is not workable for those with cognitive impairment or who suffer periods of confusion. This scenario is likely to end in further confusion and poor compliance. A familiar face or set of care workers is always going to be the most effective team and in whom the patient has most faith. Underlying all these principles is communication.

Communication

Establishing good lines of communication between the various strands of health care is often very challenging. In palliative care the aim is to utilize these lines of communication to ensure the patient and loved ones are central to this process. Part of this centrality includes the rights of the patient to partake in decision-making, and once again this may involve the relatives, partner or loved ones. An example of this may be deciding where to die, should a real choice exist, and here loved ones may need to shoulder the burden of care if dying at home is a viable option.

CONCLUSION

The case of A.S. has most probably been repeated many times over in all areas of the world, since the epidemic of HIV began to unfold in the early 1980s.

We believe the features which enabled him to rehabilitate and resettle in his community were many, not least his individual determination to do just that, that is, to leave hospital.

Other factors are worth mentioning – for example, the aim to listen to his desires and wishes was prominent. Attempting to integrate services, and ensuring co-operation between statutory and voluntary services were also important.

The availability of specialized services in the city of London was another factor, in this case to provide residential palliative care.

All in all, the multidisciplinary collaboration which effectively met the various needs of A.S. throughout his illness was testament to the commitment of all concerned.

Further reading

Adler, M.W. (ed.) *ABC of AIDS*, British Medical Publications, London, 1987.

BMA Foundation for AIDS. *The Management of HIV Infection in Primary Care*. British Medical Association Foundation for AIDS, London, 1990.

Cohen, P.T., Sande, M.A. and Volberding, P.A. (eds) *The AIDS Knowledge Base*, The Medical Publishing Group, Waltham, MA, 1990.

Farthing, C., Brown, S. and Staughton, R. *A Colour Atlas of AIDS and HIV Disease* (2nd edition), Wolfe Publishing Ltd, London, 1988.

Frontliners. *Living with AIDS: A guide to survival by people with AIDS*, Frontliners, London, 1987.

HIV and Human Rights – From Victim to Victor, The Voice of People with HIV and AIDS. (1991) Report of the Fifth International Conference for People with HIV and AIDS.

Kübler-Ross, E. *AIDS: the Ultimate Challenge*, MacMillan, New York, 1987.

Kübler-Ross, E. *Living with death and dying*. Souvenir Press, London, 1982.

Miller, R. and Bor, R. *AIDS: A guide to clinical counselling*, Science Press, London, 1988.

Moss, A. *HIV and AIDS: Management by the primary care team*, Oxford University Press, Oxford, 1992.

Newbury, J. and Walsh, J. *Looking After People With Late HIV Disease*, Patten Press in Association with the Lisa Sainbury Foundation Publisher, London, 1990.

O'Sullivan, S. and Thomson, K. *Living with AIDS*, Sheba Feminist Press, London, 1992.

Pratt, R. *AIDS: A strategy for Nursing Care* (3rd edition), Edward Arnold, London, 1991.

Richardson, A. and Bolle, D. *Wise Before Their Time: People Living with AIDS and HIV*, Harper Collins, London, 1992.

Richardson, D. *Women and AIDS and Society*, Pandora Press, London, 1987.

Robertson, R. *Heroin, AIDS and Society*, Hodder and Stoughton, London, 1987.

Royal College of Nursing. *AIDS: Nursing Guidelines*, Royal College of Nursing, 20 Cavendish Square, London W1M 0AAB, 1986.

Scott, P. *National AIDS Manual*, National AIDS Manual Press, London, 1988.

Shilts, R. *And The Band Played On*, Penguin Books, Harmondsworth, 1988.

Sims, R. and Moss, V. *Terminal Care for People with AIDS*, Edward Arnold, London, 1991.

Yelding, D. *Caring for Someone with AIDS*. Research Institute for Consumer Affairs and Disabilities Study Unit. Hodder and Stoughton, London, 1990.

Youle, M., *et al. AIDS: Therapeutics in HIV Disease*, Churchill Livingstone, Edinburgh, 1988.

Appendix

Acute Regimes

Condition under treatment	Medication	Regime	Adverse effects
Respiratory System Pulmonary Tuberculosis	Rifampicin	Daily	Rashes, fevers, nausea, vomiting, orange, red discoloration of secretions, i.e. tears/urine
	Ethambutol	Daily	Nausea, vomiting eyes, colour blindness visual disturbance
	Isoniazid	Daily	Peripheral neuritis fevers liver dysfunction
Vit B6 prevents some of the adverse effects of the Isonazid, i.e. peripheral neuritis	Pyridoxine (Vitamin B6)	Daily	
Pulmonary TB where quadruple therapy is necessary	Pyrazinamide	Daily	Rashes, joint pains nausea, vomiting

*All medications are oral unless otherwise stated

Prophylactic Regimes

Condition under treatment	Medication	Regime	Adverse effects
Pneumocystis carinii pneumonia (PCP)	Co-trimoxazole (Contains two antibiotics Sulphamethoxazole & Trimethoprim)	Daily/alternate days	Rashes nausea, vomiting, anaemia general malaise Stevens-Johnson's syndrome
	Dapsone/Trimethoprim	Daily	Rashes nausea, vomiting abnormal liver function anaemia
	Pentamidine usually via a nebulizer	Bi-monthly	Rashes intolerance of nebulizer mask malaise, cough, wheezing hyperglycaemia, hypoglycaemia abnormal kidney function diarrhoea
Gastrointestinal system			
Candida (Thrush)	Nystan, Amphotericin lozenges or mouth washes Nystan Pessaries	Up to 4 hours/ Daily	Few adverse effects noted though nausea, vomiting, diarrhoea
	Ketoconazole	Daily	Nausea, vomiting liver dysfunction
	Itraconazole	Daily	Nausea, vomiting
	Fluconazole	Daily	Nausea, vomiting
Herpes Simplex/Zoster	Acyclovir	Daily	Few adverse effects noted nausea, vomiting, diarrhoea

contd

Prophylactic Regimes

Condition under treatment	Medication	Regime	Adverse effects
Nervous system			
Toxoplasmosis	Fansidar (contains two antibiotics: Pyrimethamine with Sulphadoxine)	Daily	Rashes nausea, vomiting anaemia, abdominal discomfort kidney dysfunction, headache
Cytomegalovirus (CMV)	Ganciclovir • Intravenous treatment usual • Requires special monitoring	Daily (5–7 days/week)	Nausea, vomiting anaemia, liver dysfunction oedema bone marrow suppression
	Foscarnet • Intravenous treatment usual • Requires special monitoring	Daily (5–7 days/week)	Nausea, vomiting anaemia, kidney dysfunction calcium dysfunction headaches

*All medications are oral unless otherwise stated

Other Regimes

Condition under treatment	Medication	Regime	Adverse effects
General conditions			
Pain	Aspirin	4 Hourly	Allergies, intolerance sweating gastric irritation
	Paracetamol	4 Hourly	Adverse effects rare: intolerance rashes
	Codeine	4 Hourly	Nausea, vomiting constipation
	Morphine	4 Hourly	Nausea, vomiting constipation, respiratory depression somnolence, tiredness
Lack of appetite	Megestrol	Daily	Occasional rashes nausea, vomiting impotence
Space occupying lesion within cranium ⎫ Raised Intra-Cranial Pressure ⎬ Lack of Appetite ⎭	Dexamethasone	Daily	Gastric irritation May trigger peptic ulceration disinhibition and euphoria occasional psychosis
HIV Infection	Zidovudine (AZT)	Daily	Nausea, vomiting rashes, muscle pains/headaches anaemia
HIV Infection	Dideoxyinosine (DDI)	Daily	Nausea, vomiting electrolyte disturbances pancreatitis neuropathy

*All medications are oral unless otherwise stated

Index

Page numbers appearing in **bold** refer to figures and page numbers appearing in *italic* refer to tables.